D0782083

BASIC CONCEPTS *IN*

Neuroscience

A STUDENT'S SURVIVAL GUIDE

BASIC CONCEPTS

IN

Neuroscience

A STUDENT'S SURVIVAL GUIDE

Editor

MALCOLM SLAUGHTER, PhD

Department of Physiology and Biophysics
State University of New York at Buffalo
Buffalo, New York

Illustrated by

JOHN NYQUIST, MS, CMI

BARBARA E. EVANS, BFA

Medical Illustrations and Graphics, ASCIT
State University of New York at Buffalo
Buffalo, New York

McGraw-Hill
Medical Publishing Division

New York   Chicago   San Francisco
Lisbon   London   Madrid
Mexico City   Milan   New Delhi   San Juan
Seoul   Singapore   Sydney   Toronto

McGraw-Hill

A Division of The McGraw·Hill Companies

**BASIC CONCEPTS IN NEUROSCIENCE:
A STUDENT'S SURVIVAL GUIDE**

Copyright © 2002 by **The McGraw-Hill Companies, Inc.** All rights reserved. Printed in the United States of America. Except as permitted under the United States Copyright Act of 1976, no part of this publication may be reproduced or distributed in any form or by any means, or stored in a data base or retrieval system, without the prior written permission of the publisher.

1 2 3 4 5 6 7 8 9 0 DOC DOC 0 9 8 7 6 5 4 3 2 1

ISBN 0-07-136046-8

This book was set in Times Roman by V&M Graphics, Inc.
The editors were Janet Foltin, Harriet Lebowitz, and Lester A. Sheinis.
The series editor was Hiram F. Gilbert, PhD.
The production supervisor was Richard C. Ruzycka.
The cover designer was Mary McDonnell.
The indexer was Alexandra Nickerson.

R. R. Donnelley & Sons Company was printer and binder.

This book is printed on acid-free paper.

Library of Congress Cataloging-in-Publication Data

Basic concepts in neuroscience: a student's survival guide / edited by Malcolm Slaughter.—1st ed.
    p. ; cm.
  ISBN 0-07-136046-8 (alk. paper)
  1. Neurosciences. 2. Neurobiology. I. Slaughter, Malcolm.
[DNLM: 1. Nervous System—Handbooks. WL 39 B311 2001]
QP355.2. B37 2001
612.8—dc21   2001031229

INTERNATIONAL EDITION ISBN 0-07-112016-5
Copyright © 2002. Exclusive rights by The McGraw-Hill Companies, Inc., for manufacture and export. This book cannot be reexported from the country to which it is consigned by McGraw-Hill. The International Edition is not available in North America.

Dedicated to Dr. Beverly Bishop, Distinguished Professor of Physiology and Biophysics, for her tireless and timely support of neuroscience at the University of Buffalo

· C O N T E N T S ·

CHAPTER 4 SYNAPTIC TRANSMISSION 65
Edward Koenig

CHAPTER 5 NEUROTRANSMITTERS 86
Jerome Roth

CHAPTER 6 SENSORY SYSTEMS 117
Malcolm Slaughter

· C O N T R I B U T O R S ·

John M. Aletta, PhD
Clinical Assistant Professor of Pharmacology
   and Toxicology
Department of Pharmacology and Toxicology
State University of New York at Buffalo
Buffalo, New York
Chapter 2

Beverly P. Bishop, PhD
Professor of Physiology and Biophysics
Department of Physiology and Biophysics
University at Buffalo
State University of New York
Buffalo, New York
Chapters 7, 8, 9

Kathleen M.K. Boje, PhD
Associate Professor of Pharmaceutics
Department of Pharmaceutics, School of
   Pharmacy
State University of New York at Buffalo
Buffalo, New York
Chapter 12

Arlene R. Collins, MA, PhD
Professor of Microbiology
Department of Microbiology, School of
   Medicine and Biomedical Sciences
State University of New York at Buffalo
Buffalo, New York
Chapter 13

Dennis M. Higgins, PhD
Professor of Pharmacology and Toxicology
Department of Pharmacology and Toxicology
State University of New York at Buffalo
Buffalo, New York
Chapter 1

Elaine M. Hull, PhD
Professor of Psychology
Department of Psychology
State University of New York at Buffalo
Buffalo, New York
Chapter 10

Edward Koenig, PhD
Professor of Physiology and Biophysics
Department of Physiology and Biophysics
State University of New York at Buffalo
Buffalo, New York
Chapter 4

Jerome Roth, PhD
Professor of Pharmacology and Toxicology
Department of Pharmacology and Toxicology
State University of New York at Buffalo
Buffalo, New York
Chapter 5

Malcolm Slaughter, PhD
Professor of Physiology and Biophysics
Department of Physiology and Biophysics
State University of New York at Buffalo
Buffalo, New York
Chapters 3, 6

Susan B. Udin, PhD
Professor of Physiology and Biophysics
Department of Physiology and Biophysics
State University of New York at Buffalo
Buffalo, New York
Chapter 11

· P R E F A C E ·

Basic Concepts in Neuroscience: A Student's Survival Guide is designed to provide a quick reference to the key topics in neuroscience. It is oriented toward the needs of medical, graduate, and advanced undergraduate students. Each chapter highlights the basic principles of the field, coupled with a description of experimental protocols that clarifies and amplifies the subject. Although interrelated, each chapter is intended to be self-explanatory so the student can focus on areas of interest.

This book is designed to be easily read and to quickly guide students through the fundamentals of neuroscience. The format of each chapter includes highlighted summary statements. The authors made a special effort to include many flowcharts and figures in each chapter that can serve as study guides. We recommend that students review these statements and figures to obtain an overview of the chapter. In striving for clarity, we emphasized essential principles and made brevity a virtue. We hope the reader values this approach; however, we recommend that this book be used in combination with a more extensive neuroscience textbook.

A group of faculty at the University at Buffalo wrote this book based on a graduate level course: Introduction to Neuroscience. Each chapter was written by a faculty researcher who is a specialist on the chapter topic, ensuring that the content is not only factual but also current. The goal has been to make the descriptions readable and interesting, yet to convey the excitement of the evolving science of the brain. The faculty's commitment to exposing students to research-based learning is clearly shown in the numerous examples of information imparted within an experimental framework.

I want to thank all of the faculty members who contributed to this book. It was one more obligation in an overburdened schedule, but each one contributed magnificently. Special thanks go to John Nyquist and Barbara Evans, whose drawings enliven every chapter. I am very grateful for the guidance, patience, and expertise of the editors at McGraw-Hill: Janet Foltin, Harriet Lebowitz, Lester A. Sheinis, and Arline Keithe.

BASIC CONCEPTS IN Neuroscience

A STUDENT'S SURVIVAL GUIDE

·C H A P T E R · 1 ·

CELL BIOLOGY OF THE NERVOUS SYSTEM

·

Dennis M. Higgins

Specialized Adaptations of Neurons

Glia and Other Nonneuronal Cells

· · · · · · · · · · · ·

The two most important types of cells within the nervous system are *neurons* and *glia*. These cells are specialized to perform three basic functions: to receive information from the five senses, to integrate these data, and to generate motor behaviors that ensure the survival of the organism.

To accomplish these tasks, neurons and glia have acquired specialized properties that facilitate the processing of information. The unique cellular characteristics of neurons are the most obvious and most important.

1

Confusing terminology. Neuron and *nerve cell* are synonyms that refer to the major information-conveying cells in the nervous system. *Neural cell,* however, refers to all of the cells in the nervous system, including both neurons and glia. *Nerve* refers to long projections that emanate from the central nervous system. Typically nerves contain axons and glia but not the cell bodies of nerve cells.

SPECIALIZED ADAPTATIONS OF NEURONS

What happens when you step on a sharp object? First a signal must be conveyed from the foot to the spinal cord and higher brain centers (Figure 1–1) indicating the presence of a painful stimulus; the motor neurons must then stimulate

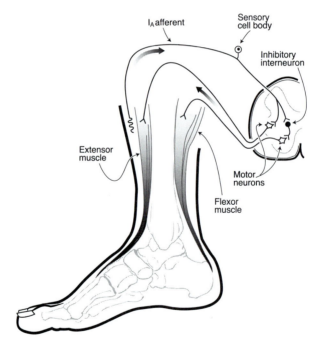

Figure 1–1
A simple reflex. Painful stimuli are detected by nerve terminals in the skin and parenchyma. Pain and pressure are converted by the nerve into electrical signals that are propagated along the sensory nerve toward the spinal cord. These impulses are then transmitted across synaptic junctions to cause excitation of motor neurons, which in turn causes the contraction of distal muscles.

the muscles, causing the foot to be lifted. To accomplish this seemingly simple task, information must be conducted over a distance of ~1 m, the distance from the foot to the spinal cord. One meter is equivalent to 1,000,000 μm. Because human cells rarely exceed 50 μm in diameter, transmission of information over this distance represents a formidable cellular challenge.

The evolutionary solution for this problem has been for neurons to acquire the ability to form long, thin processes that can bridge the entire distance from the foot to the spinal cord. These processes are called *axons*.

Axons represent only a partial solution to the problem of information transfer over long distances; for the system to function properly other specializations are needed. To allow the organism to respond to environmental changes in a timely manner, information has to be conveyed rapidly from one end of the axon to the other. This requirement is met by the electrical propagation of signals along the axon (see Chapter 3). In addition, information must be conveyed in a polarized manner, that is, it must proceed from the sensory neuron to the spinal cord and then to the motor neuron.

The specialized cellular junctions that direct this information flow are called *synapses*.

These are described in more detail in Chapter 4.

Although the axon represents an elegant solution to the problem of conveying information over long distances, this cellular adaptation comes with a significant cost. Axons typically have diameters ranging from 0.2 to 10 μm, and the cell body of neurons is typically ~20 μm in diameter. To obtain some idea of what this means in terms of asymmetry, consider Figure 1–2, which shows the neuronal cell body with a 20-mm diameter, that is, at a 1000-fold magnification of a neuron that is 20 μm in diameter, and the axon's diameter at 1000-fold magnification. However, at this scale only a small fragment of the axon's initial length is shown, because to show the 1,000,000-μm length of the axon the figure would have to be 1,000,000 mm long. This is equivalent to 1 km. Thus, if the axon terminal was drawn to scale, it would require a piece of paper about 0.6 miles long.

How does this extreme asymmetry affect the nerve cell? Imagine what would happen if you tried to extend a piece of steel wire for a half mile between two high buildings. It would sag under its own weight and then break.

Figure 1–2

Dimensions of a sensory neuron. Sensory neurons typically have only one axon that bifurcates shortly after leaving the cell body (only one branch is shown to simplify the diagram). The axon is a narrow cylinder (~1–5 μm in diameter) that extends for long distances. For example, the axons of some sensory neurons have one branch that goes to the large toe and another branch that goes to the brain, a total distance of about 2,000,000 μm. The cell body and axon are drawn to scale with 1 mm representing 1 μm.

Thus the extreme length of the axon poses structural problems that require both cytoskeletal specializations and interactions with glia and other matrix-producing cells.

In addition, there are metabolic problems. Axons are exceedingly narrow tubes, and macromolecules do not move well by diffusion along such structures. Most of the proteins and vesicular components required for the function and maintenance of axons are made in the neuronal cell body. Thus, specialized mechanisms of rapid transport are required to maintain an adequate supply of axonal proteins; however, even with this specialization, they remain under substantial metabolic strain. That is one of the reasons that peripheral neuropathies are commonly associated with metabolic disorders.

Parts of a Neuron

Neurons that subserve different functions have different shapes. Sensory neurons are among the simplest in terms of structure. They have a cell body and a single axonal process that conducts information from peripheral structures to the central nervous system. Most other neurons have two types of processes that arise from their cell body.

> The most common configuration is *multiple dendrites* and a *single axon* (Figure 1–3). In such cells, the dendrites function as afferent or receptive processes, whereas the axon is the efferent process that conveys signals to the target cells.

For example, in the case of the motor neuron, its many dendrites receive afferent information from the brain and sensory fibers, which is then integrated in the cell body and sent out along the axon to muscle fibers. Thus, as in the case of sensory fibers, information in motor fibers flows in a polarized fashion from the dendrites to the soma and out along the axon.

The Neuronal Cell Body

> The *neuronal cell body,* also known as the *soma* or *perikaryon,* has all the organelles found in other cells, including a nucleus, Golgi apparatus, and smooth and rough endoplasmic reticulum.

Almost all of the proteins destined for axons and most of the dendritic proteins are made in the soma. Because of this heavy anabolic requirement, neurons generally have an abundance of rough endoplasmic reticulum and many polysomes. The nucleic acids present in ribosomes of the endoplasmic reticulum and polysomes react strongly with aniline dyes such as cresyl violet and toluidine, and so neurons exhibit prominent staining with these agents. The stained material is commonly referred to as *Nissl substance.* Because of the high rates of protein synthesis, neuronal chromatin is typically dispersed and nucleoli are prominent. The proteins made by neurons are exceedingly diverse, and it is estimated that more than 50% of the genome is expressed in the brain.

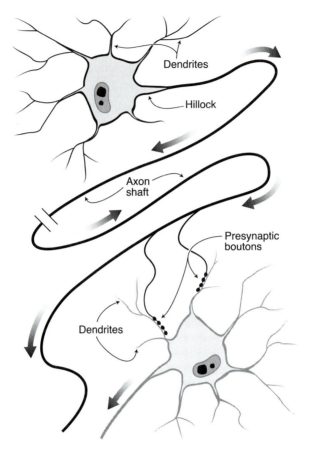

Figure 1–3
Parts of a neuron. Most neurons are multipolar cells having one axon and several dendrites. Information flows in a polarized manner in these cells (*arrows*). Typically incoming signals are received in the dendrites and they proceed through the cell body to the axon hillock where they are integrated. Efferent signals are conducted down the axonal shaft, through the terminal branches, and into the presynaptic boutons. There they elicit the release of neurotransmitters.

Neural stem cells, capable of dividing and giving rise to new neurons, persist in some parts of the adult mammalian nervous system, and they are particularly prominent in the olfactory epithelium. However, most neurons become postmitotic at about the time of birth. Thus, to a first approximation, mammals have the maximum complement of neurons early in life, and neurons that are lost to disease, injury, or aging are not replaced. To compensate for the lack of replacements, most neurons have a spare metabolic capacity. Thus, when a fraction of a neuronal cell population is lost, the remaining cells hypertrophy and assume the former load of the dead cells. The clinical consequence of this spare capacity is that neurological symptoms in degenerative conditions such as Parkinson disease do not usually become apparent until there has been a loss of 70% or more of the relevant population of neurons. Another consequence of the long life of neural cells is that many of them gradually accumulate deposits of lipofuscin and other cellular debris.

Dendrites

> *Dendrites* are the afferent part of the neuron that is specialized for receiving signals.

One of their functions is to increase the surface area of the neuron available for synapse formation. However, dendrites also facilitate the orderly flow and processing of information. For example, in some cases auditory and visual inputs are processed by different dendrites; in other cases, information from various brain regions is allocated to specific dendritic domains. Thus dendrites are not merely passive structures that simply amplify the receptive surface; rather they are also involved in the active integration of afferent information.

The Axon

> Neurons typically have only one *axon,* which has three parts: hillock, shaft, and terminal.

The initial segment of the axon is called the *hillock,* the site at which electrical signals are integrated within the cells (see Chapter 3). Synapses are often formed on this part of the neuron. The hillock is the region at which the cytoplasm of the soma funnels down to the narrow opening of the axon and cytoskeletal elements become aligned. Organelles such as the Golgi apparatus and rough endoplasmic reticulum are blocked from entry into the hillock, and it is thought that much of the sorting of cytoplasmic constituents occurs in this region.

The axon *shaft,* a long, thin cylindrical tube of uniform diameter, is specialized for conducting electrical signals and for transporting material to the axon terminal. The shaft typically lacks synaptic contacts. In mature mammals, the various types of axons either lack the ability or have a very limited capacity to make proteins, and this is reflected in a paucity of polyribosomes and rough endoplasmic reticulum. The axonal cytoplasm is, however, enriched in cytoskeletal elements, including intermediate filaments, microtubules, and microfilaments (Figure 1–4). These are typically oriented as parallel arrays following the long axis of the axonal shaft.

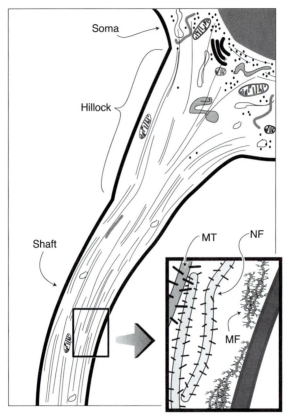

Figure 1–4
Structure of the axon. The main duties of the axon shaft are to conduct electrical
impulses and to transport material to and from the axon terminals. Therefore, the axonal
shaft typically contains large numbers of filaments and limited numbers of organelles,
with exclusion of the latter beginning in the hillock region. *Inset*: Microtubules (MT)
and neurofilaments (NF) tend to be aligned in parallel arrays within the core of the
axon. In contrast, bundles of actin-containing microfilaments (MF) are more common
in cortical regions where they frequently contact the plasma membrane. Vesicular
components are typically transported along microtubules.

Distinctions Between Axons and Dendrites

There are profound differences in the morphological properties of dendrites and axons.

1. Most neurons have multiple dendrites but only one axon.
2. The dendritic cytoplasm is initially continuous with the somatic cytoplasm and lacks a hillock-like region.
3. Dendrites typically branch near the soma and end locally, whereas the axon typically travels long distances before it begins branching.
4. Dendrites are tapered in contrast to axons, which have a cylindrical shape.
5. Dendrites branch at Y-shaped angles, whereas axonal collaterals may arise at right or even obtuse angles.

These differences in axonal and dendritic shape and morphology probably arise from differences in their cytoskeletal composition, including the dendritic enrichment in microtubule-associated protein 2 (MAP2), and the random orientation of their microtubules.

> Dendrites also have a distinct membrane composition. They are different from axons, having more receptor-activated ion channels and fewer voltage-activated channels.

They also have a distinct endosomal pathway. Typically the dendritic plasma membrane is composed of small synaptic mosaics (Figure 1–5), with each region displaying the unique specializations required to accommodate the opposing type of presynaptic axons. Thus, the membrane underlying neurons that release acetylcholine needs to be different from the membrane underlying neurons that use glutamate as their neurotransmitter. One of the major current problems in neuroscience is understanding how these thousands of small microdomains are established and maintained.

The Neuronal Cytoskeleton

Neurofilaments

> *Neurofilaments,* a form of intermediate filament found only in neurons, are long linear polymers composed of three proteins: the heavy (200 kDa), medium (160 kDa), and low (70 kDa) subunits.

Neurofilaments are more prominent in large axons and less prominent in dendrites and small-diameter fibers. Axonal neurofilaments contain more phosphate groups than dendritic neurofilaments, and this posttranslational modification appears to occur primarily in the axonal shaft. Neurofilaments are the most stable and least dynamic cytoskeletal constituents of neurons. They are thought to pro-

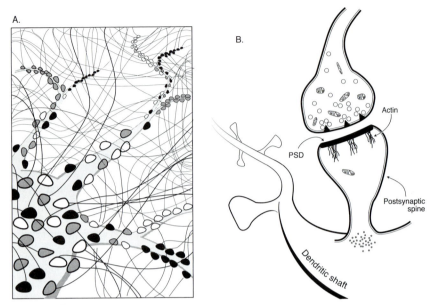

Figure 1–5
Synaptic contacts. (**A**) The neuronal surface is covered with numerous synaptic contacts
(up to 100,000/neuron). Synapses are most prominent on dendrites but also occur on
the soma and axon hillock. Numerous types of axons contact neurons and many use
different neurotransmitters (varying gray tones). For efficient transmission, the postsynaptic membranes must form a mosaic patchwork with proper receptors inserted
below each of the different types of axons. (**B**) The axon terminal contains numerous
synaptic vesicles, some of which are associated with membranous release sites. The
postsynaptic cell typically has a postsynaptic density (PSD) that contains receptors and
ion channels that are associated with cytoskeletal fibers. Ribosomes (dots) are frequently
found at the base of spines.

vide much of the mechanical strength of axons and the spacing of their sidearms,
and their phosphate groups are an important determinant of axonal diameter.

Microtubules   Microtubules are also a prominent constituent of axons; indeed,
the proteins associated with these structures represent ~5% of the entire protein
content of the brain. Axonal microtubules can be exceptionally long, sometimes
attaining lengths of several hundred microns. As in other cells, neuronal microtubules are composed of polymerized α- and β-tubulin subunits that are complexed with a large number of MAPs that regulate their stability and assembly.
However, axonal microtubules have two unique characteristics.

Microtubules are polarized.

They have both a *plus* end at which tubulin subunits are added to the polymer and a *minus* end at which depolymerization occurs. Axonal microtubules have a unique polarity with all of the plus ends being oriented away from the cell body and the minus ends facing the soma. In this respect they differ from dendritic microtubules, which have a random distribution of about half the plus ends facing the soma and the remainder facing the other direction.

> Axonal microtubules are also distinguished by their high content of the MAP called tau and their lack of MAP2.

In this respect, they are also clearly different from dendrites that are enriched in MAP2 and deficient in tau. There are also differences in the degree of phosphorylation of tau in axons and dendrites. The cytoskeletal differences between axons and dendrites are thought to underlie the basic differences in the shape and branching patterns of these processes. Currently there is much interest in the biology of tau because it is the primary constituent of the paired helical filaments that are present in the neuritic tangles that are characteristic of Alzheimer disease.

Microtubules and Neuronal Transport

> Microtubules contribute to the mechanical strength of axons. They are also involved in *fast axonal transport.*

As previously mentioned, the axon is so narrow that it would require decades for proteins to move from the soma to the nerve terminal by diffusion. Therefore, active transport mechanisms are required. The fastest rates of axonal transport are observed with vesicular components, such as synaptic vesicles and mitochondria. These organelles move at rates of ~200–400 mm/day, meaning that material made in the cell body can reach the axon terminals within a few days. Fast axonal transport requires both microtubules and microtubule motor proteins. The latter proteins are adenosine triphosphatases (ATPases), which have binding sites for both microtubules and vesicles; the hydrolysis of adenosine triphosphate (ATP) is used to propel the vesicle along the microtubule. Several motor proteins belonging to the kinesin family move vesicular material along the microtubule in a polarized manner from the minus end to the plus end; these are strong candidates for being the motors that convey material from the soma to the nerve terminals. This is called *anterograde transport.*

Neurons also have a fast transport mechanism for moving vesicular material in the opposite direction: from the nerve terminal to the cell body. This is called *retrograde transport.* Classes of proteins moved in this manner include nerve growth factors and their receptors. These growth-inducing proteins convey important information to the nucleus about the state of the axon terminals. For example, between birth and adulthood, the growth of the animal is accompanied by an enormous increase in the surface area of the skin. To maintain a constant density of sensory endings within the skin, it is necessary for the nerve terminals to grow into the newly formed tissue. This type of neural sprouting is induced by trophic factors that are secreted by the targets of sensory neurons and then transported back to the soma. Microtubule motors that move proteins from the plus to the minus end of microtubules are responsible for retrograde transport; one of the most important appears to be dynein.

> Fast anterograde and retrograde transport move only vesicular cellular components. Nonvesicular materials, such as microtubules, neurofilaments, and cytoplasmic enzymes, move down the axon at a much slower rate (2–5 mm/day).

The cellular basis of this movement is not well understood, and, indeed, because the various nonvesicular components move at varying rates, several different mechanisms may be involved. However, the slowness of the transport has important clinical consequences. A transport rate of 5 mm/day means that material made in the spinal cord will require more than 200 days to reach the nerve terminal 1 m, or 1000 mm, away. This is one of the reasons that recovery from peripheral neuropathies can be quite slow, requiring 6 months to 1 year.

Microfilaments   Microfilaments are found throughout the neuron, but they are particularly prominent in the axonal cortex just below the plasma membrane.

> Microfilaments are polymers of β- and γ-actin that typically are associated with contractile proteins, including nonmuscle myosins, and a variety of proteins regulating actin polymerization.

The latter include factors involved in actin binding, capping, nucleation, and severing. Microfilaments play a prominent role in proper positioning and anchoring of membrane proteins such as ion channels and receptors. They are also involved in the growth and guidance of axons during development.

The Synapse

The axon shaft, on reaching its target, begins to branch and send off collaterals. These daughter processes then form synapses, often giving rise to hundreds or thousands of contacts.

> *Synapses* are cellular junctions designed to convey information in a polarized fashion from a neuron to its target cell (see Figure 1–5). Synapses usually involve two cells: the *presynaptic* and *postsynaptic* elements.

In most cases, the presynaptic component is an axon and the postsynaptic element is a neuronal dendrite or cell body or muscle cell. Most mammalian synapses use small molecules known as neurotransmitters to convey information from the presynaptic cell to the postsynaptic cell. For this mode of transmission to be effective, axonal presynaptic elements must have specializations that facilitate the secretion of chemical neurotransmitters and the postsynaptic partner must have corresponding apparatuses that allow it to respond to the neurotransmitter.

Typical axon presynaptic specializations include the following:

1. clusters of synaptic vesicles that contain the neurotransmitter;
2. presynaptic membrane densities that represent sites for the fusion of synaptic vesicles and the subsequent exocytosis of their constituent neurotransmitters;
3. smooth endoplasmic reticulum required for vesicular biogenesis and recirculation; and
4. accumulations of mitochondria to generate the energy required for the synthesis and release of neurotransmitter.

Typical postsynaptic specializations observed in dendrites and muscle cells include the clustering of neurotransmitter receptors and their downstream signaling elements in apposition to the site transmitter release. Specific cytoplasmic proteins such as rapsyn and gephrin anchor some types of receptors to webs of microfilaments, whereas other receptors are aggregated by membrane-associated guanylate kinases (MAGUKs) and other proteins containing PDZ domains. The accumulation of membranous and perimembranous proteins at synaptic junctions gives rise to *postsynaptic densities,* that is, regions of the postsynaptic contacts that exhibit increased electron density and staining in the electron microscope.

Location of Synapses   Although a few synapses are formed on the neuronal soma and axon hillock,

> dendrites are the primary site of synapse formation in the mammalian nervous system.

Synapses are present on the dendritic shaft. In many cells, the dendrites also have tiny protrusions that arise from the shaft and exhibit postsynaptic specializations. These are called *dendritic spines,* and they can be numerous (some cells have tens of thousands of spines). Dendrites also have protein synthetic machinery, including ribosomes, and these tend to be concentrated below the synaptic structures and spines. Proteins made by these dendritic ribosomes are thought to play an important role in synaptic plasticity and learning.

GLIA AND OTHER NONNEURONAL CELLS

> *Glia* are the most numerous cell type in the nervous system. One of their most important functions is to ensheathe nerve cells and thereby provide mechanical support.

Indeed, with the exception of synaptic surfaces, the entire neuron is typically covered by a patchwork of membranous sheets made by one or more types of glial cell.

Glia in the Peripheral Nervous System

> There is only one type of glial cell in the peripheral nervous system: the *Schwann cell.*

The Schwann cell ensheathes axons in a diameter-dependent manner. If the axonal diameter is less than ~1 μm, the Schwann cell simply surrounds the axon but does not wrap around it repeatedly (Figure 1–6). In contrast, if the process diameter exceeds 1 μm, the Schwann cell typically invests the axon with multiple wraps or layers of membrane that contain specialized membrane proteins and lipids. This insulating investment of the axon by the Schwann cell is called *myelin,* and it enhances the capacity of the axon to conduct electrical signals (Chapter 3). In the peripheral nervous system, the neuronal soma and dendrites are also ensheathed by glia. The specialized type of Schwann cell that covers these parts of the neuron is usually referred to as a satellite cell.

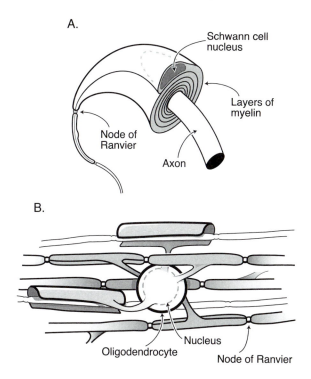

Figure 1–6

Myelination of axons. Glia cover all the surfaces of a neuron, including axons, dendrites, cell bodies, and synapses. Large-diameter axons receive a specialized form of ensheathement called myelin. This lipid-rich investment insulates the axon and facilitates the conduction of electrical impulses. Myelin segments are typically ~1 mm in length and are separated by openings called nodes of Ranvier. In the peripheral nervous system (**A**), a single myelin segment is made by one Schwann cell whose membrane repeatedly wraps around the axon. In the central nervous system (**B**), myelin is made by oligodendrocytes. These cells extend multiple processes, each of which can form a myelin segment.

In addition to providing mechanical support and ensheathement, Schwann cells also make neurotrophic factors and provide a surface that supports axonal growth.

These properties enhance recovery of peripheral nerve after injury. The powerful trophic support provided by Schwann cells is responsible for much of the regenerative capacity of the peripheral nervous system. In contrast, glia in the mature central nervous system do not appear to provide the same level of trophic support and do not allow the same degree of regeneration.

Peripheral nerve also contains other types of nonneuronal cells including *fibroblasts, macrophages,* and *mast cells.* The fibroblasts produce collagen I, elastin, and other connective tissue proteins that give peripheral nerve its great tensile strength.

Glia in the Central Nervous System

The population of nonneuronal cells in the central nervous system differs from that in the peripheral nervous system in the following ways:

1. The central nervous system lacks fibroblasts and so it does not contain typical extracellular matrix proteins such as collagens and elastins.
2. The only phagocytic cell normally present in the brain is the microglial cell. Macrophages and neutrophils appear only after injury or inflammation.
3. The central nervous system lacks Schwann cells, which are replaced by the macroglia.

There are two types of macroglia: *oligodendrocytes* and *astrocytes.*

Oligodendrocytes are the myelin-producing cell of the central nervous system. They are functionally similar to Schwann cells in that they invest only large-diameter axons. However, oligodendrocytes differ from Schwann cells: oligodendrocytes are capable of making multiple myelin segments, whereas a Schwann cell can produce only one myelin segment.

Astrocytes are typically subdivided into two classes: *fibrous* and *protoplasmic.*

Fibrous astrocytes are more prominent in white matter and contain high concentrations of glial fibrillary acid protein (GFAP), a form of intermediate filament found only in glia. Protoplasmic astrocytes are more common in gray matter and have lower concentrations of GFAP. Both types of astrocyte ensheathe the small-diameter axons that are not contacted by oligodendrocytes, and they cover the soma and dendrites. Astrocytes also form specialized contacts with the endothelial cells that line the capillaries in the brain. These endothelial contacts are called *glial end feet* and are thought to facilitate the transport of bloodborne nutrients to neurons.

Astrocytes perform several other important functions within the brain. Astrocytes help to maintain ionic homeostasis by buffering the cations released during prolonged neural stimulation, and they assist in the inactivation of certain neurotransmitters, including glutamate and γ-aminobutyric acid. Astrocytes also divide after injury to fill the spaces left by dead neurons, and they provide some trophic support for neurons. However, this is usually not sufficient to sustain significant regeneration after brain injury in adults.

Finally, astrocytes influence the behavior of the endothelial cells in the brain and cause them to form large numbers of tight junctions. Thus, the capillaries in the brain are significantly less permeable than those in other tissues of the body, and they prevent the diffusion of either high-molecular-weight or highly charged molecules from blood to brain. Thus, astrocytes cause endothelial cells to erect the blood–brain barrier. Clinically, this is important because the blood–brain barrier prevents many drugs from reaching the brain. This may be either an impediment (for example, getting an antibiotic to the brain to treat meningitis) or an asset (for example, avoiding potential central nervous system complications of an administered protein).

· C H A P T E R · 2 ·

DEVELOPMENTAL BIOLOGY OF THE NERVOUS SYSTEM

·

John M. Aletta

Introduction

Neural Induction

Cellular Differentiation

Cell Migration

Process Outgrowth

Synaptogenesis and Programmed Cell Death

Synaptic Remodeling and Structural Alterations

·   ·   ·   ·   ·   ·   ·   ·   ·   ·   ·   ·

INTRODUCTION

The cellular organization of the nervous system is directly responsible for achieving the awesome functional integration of the brain, which Sir Charles Sherrington referred to as "an enchanted loom" of millions of flashing electrochemical connections. This chapter provides an introduction to the fascinating investigation of the molecular mechanisms that are responsible for the generation of the gross and fine morphological structures of the nervous system. These mechanisms are of fundamental importance in the production and maintenance of the many different functional arrays of nerve cells within the brain. The following chapters in this volume are concerned with how neurons work within integrated functional units.

Three principles form the foundations of developmental biology of the vertebrate nervous system (see numbered boxed statements).

> 1. Molecular signal transduction is of fundamental importance for the expression of cell type–specific properties.

The principal stages in the development of the nervous system are listed in Table 2–1. The molecular instructions that cause each of these stages to develop depend on biochemically defined elements of signal transduction. These include soluble *extracellular ligands* (signaling proteins secreted by all cells), *receptors* (cell membrane proteins that bind ligands with high affinity), and *intracellular transducers* (which transfer information from the cell membrane receptors to the nucleus of the cell). In some cases, insoluble ligands (*extracellular matrix*) or *cell–cell contact* can serve to trigger the receptor activation of signal transduction. This flow of information from sources outside the cell, through the cell membrane, and into the nuclear machinery of sensitive cells results in the activation and/or the deactivation of specific genes. This sequence of events permits the cell to assume the appropriate functional properties for that particular stage of development.

Table 2–1   PRINCIPAL STAGES OF NERVOUS SYSTEM DEVELOPMENT

1. Neural induction
2. Cellular differentiation
3. Cell migration
4. Process outgrowth
5. Synaptogenesis and programmed cell death
6. Synaptic remodeling and structural alterations

2. Development of the nervous system is part of the larger phenomenon of embryogenesis.

Many of the principles involved in the determination of different cell types during embryonic development are, no doubt, similar to the principles involved in neuronal development. From the fertilization of a single ovum by an individual sperm cell comes the generation of a remarkable and marvelous diversity of cell types. In the central and peripheral nervous systems the wide diversity of cell types (still poorly classified in the case of neurons) is greater than the diversity in any other organ of the human body. The analysis of *stem cells,* the earliest precursors of specific cell types, thus promises to be a very exciting undertaking in neurobiology.

3. Developmental neurobiology is the study of the entire life history of the nervous system.

There is evidence of synaptic remodeling well into adulthood. The structure and function of the nervous system can be altered by learning and experience and also by injury and disease. In some instances, these alterations appear to recapitulate developmental processes. Thus, cellular and molecular explanations of the development of nerve cells hold the keys to progress in the medical treatment of a wide variety of brain disorders as well as developmental abnormalities.

NEURAL INDUCTION

Early Events

Induction is the initiation of a fundamental change in the properties of embryonic tissue.

Fertilization of the oocyte by the sperm activates metabolic activity and DNA synthesis, resulting in replication of the genetic information from both the male and female chromosomes on a common mitotic spindle. The first cell division results in a two-cell-stage diploid *zygote.* Further cycles of cell division, which proceed asynchronously, increase the number of daughter cells known as *blastomeres* at this early stage (Figure 2–1A). This small cell aggregate is known as a

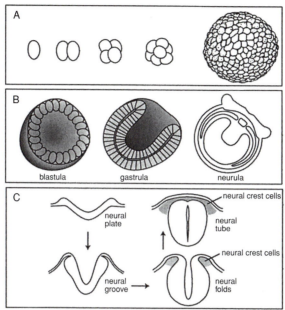

Figure 2–1
Early embryogenesis. (**A**) Formation of the morula by asynchronous cell division.
(**B**) Cross-sections of the blastula, gastrula, and neurula stages of embryonic
development. (**C**) Neurulation, the formation of the neural tube and neural crest cells.

morula (Latin = mulberry). As the cells of the morula continue to proliferate, a hollow sphere of several thousand cells is formed. This is the *blastula* (Figure 2–1B).

> Three different germ layers take shape at the end of this stage of development: ectoderm, mesoderm, and endoderm.

Ectoderm gives rise to skin, sense organs, and the nervous system. Mesoderm produces skeleton, muscle, and kidney, among other tissues. Endoderm is responsible for generation of the gastrointestinal tract.

Later Events

Ectoderm is derived from the thin cap of the blastula and endoderm from the yolk-rich cells at the thicker, vegetal pole (Figure 2–2). Induction of mesoderm, derived from ectoderm, requires an inducer or inductor from vegetal cells of the equatorial zone of the blastula.

> The ability of cells in a specific location to respond to an inducer is referred to as *competence*.

After the induction of the mesoderm germ layer, the blastula begins to fold inward at the blastopore to produce the gastrula.

Neural induction was discovered by Hilde Mangold and Hans Spemann while studying the embryonic development of amphibians.

> The onset of neural development, referred to as primary neural induction, is induced at the early gastrula stage by mesodermal cells located dorsal to a surface structure called the blastopore lip.

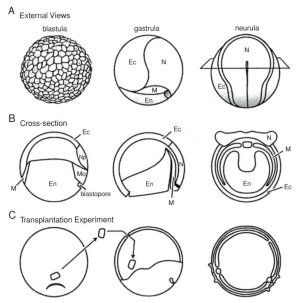

Figure 2–2
Germ layers and neural induction. External (**A**) and cross-sectional views (**B**) of the blastula, gastrula, and neurula. Ec, ectoderm; N, neural ectoderm; M, mesoderm; En, endoderm; Np, prospective neural ectoderm; Mo, mesodermal organizer region. (**C**) Transplantation of Spemann's mesodermal organizer region from just above the blastopore lip of a gastrula into ectodermal tissue of another gastrula. This results in the formation of two neural plates and, eventually, two heads complete with nervous systems.

The induced region, known as the prospective neural ectoderm, continues to proliferate and to form the neural plate (Figure 2–1C) as the embryo grows throughout gastrulation. After completion of gastrulation, the embryo progresses to the *neurula* stage (Figure 2–1B), and organogenesis, including that of the brain, begins. The neural plate increases in complexity and invaginates to form the neural groove and then the neural folds. Finally, the edges of the neural folds fuse together forming the neural tube, which has a hollow center. This structure will eventually contain cerebrospinal fluid and correspond to the lateral and third ventricles of the brain and the central canal of the spinal cord.

> The biological construction of the longitudinal closed tube of the central nervous system is called *neurulation.*

Failure of the neural tube to close leads to *spina bifida,* a birth defect of varying severity. The generation of neural crest precursors at the tips of the neural folds leads to the formation of sympathetic ganglia and adrenal chromaffin cells, among other cell fates derived from the neural ectoderm.

Spemann's Organizer

Experiments by Hans Spemann, which led to a Nobel prize in 1935, elucidated when and where cells first acquire neuronal determination in the embryo. Transplantation of a small piece of mesodermal tissue, located just dorsal to the blastopore (labeled Mo in Figure 2–2B), from a blastula stage embryo into ectoderm of another blastula (Figure 2–2C) induces a second complete nervous system in addition to the one induced by the organizer of the host embryo. Grafting other mesodermal tissue cannot produce this effect.

> This portion of mesoderm has come to be called *Spemann's organizer,* because of its remarkable ability to orchestrate the transfiguration of ectoderm into nervous tissue.

If this organizer is ablated in the late blastula, the neural plate does not form. Competence for neural induction is also limited to the ectoderm of the gastrula. Ectoderm of the blastula or neurula will not respond.

Experiments that reproduced much of this phenomenon in a cell culture dish indicated that soluble substances secreted by embryonic cells are responsible for neural induction. If ectoderm is cultured alone, skin cells develop, but no neurons.

If mesoderm from Spemann's organizer is cultured in the absence of other germ layer cells, precursors of bone, muscle, and other mesodermal somites arise, but no neurons. Even cocultures of mesoderm (excluding Spemann's organizer) and ectoderm produce cells that express markers of the notochord, muscle, kidney, and blood cells, among others, but no neurons.

> Only cocultures of Spemann's organizer and ectoderm lead to the development of cells with a neuronal phenotype.

Other Organizers

As the nervous system increases in complexity during development, additional signals from other organizer cells along the presumptive neuraxis are responsible for the formation of the brain at the anterior position and the spinal cord at the posterior position of the neuraxis. A distinctive pattern is organized positionally in both the dorsoventral and anteroposterior planes. Inductive signals that produce the forebrain are different from those that are responsible for spinal cord development. Positionally specific gene expression, such as that for *homeobox genes,* contributes to pattern formation in the central nervous system (CNS).

> A similar process of induction occurs in the peripheral nervous system (PNS). This process develops from specialized ectodermal thickenings called *placodes.*

The neural crest (Figure 2–1C) may be considered a large longitudinal placode lying at the edge of the neural fold and the ectoderm. A subpopulation of neural crest cells will become the neurons of the autonomic and dorsal root ganglia. Sensory placodes (precursors of the central sense organs for light, sound, olfaction, and taste) are induced in ectodermal tissue by contact with specific parts of the neural tube. After migration away from the neural tube, nerve fibers grow back toward the segment of the central nervous system from which the placode arose.

Inducing Molecules

There are two opposing theories concerning the development of the nervous system. Induction emphasizes the importance of cell–cell interactions. In contrast, cell lineage is based on the belief that cells are destined to a certain fate, that is, a given precursor cell is destined to become a particular neuron, such as a Purkinje cell.

> Present evidence indicates that cell–cell interactions, not cell lineage, determine a neuron's final identity.

These cell–cell interactions result from receptor recognition of either extracellular matrix molecules or soluble factors. The inducing factors bind to receptors that regulate transcription factors to control specific gene expression.

The search for the molecular identities of inducing substances constitutes a very active area of research. Scores (possibly hundreds) of different soluble substances are potentially involved in induction phenomena. Among these are the following:

> fibroblast growth factor (FGF), retinoic acid (a derivative of vitamin A), and the transforming growth factor beta (TGF-β) family.

Too little or too much retinoic acid can produce development abnormalities; for example, an excess leads to spina bifida. The somewhat bewildering wealth of possible factors makes it difficult to unequivocally resolve issues of identification. For example, activin, a member of the TGF-β family, was long thought to be necessary for the induction of mesoderm, but it has been demonstrated that this is probably not true in any simple sense. The active inducing molecule responsible for the effect of Spemann's organizer is also elusive. Identification of the true neural inducer(s) is fundamentally problematic, because there are so many potential artificial inducers or activators that can neuralize ectoderm in the artificial environment of cell culture. It has become clear that most of these potential molecules are not physiologically relevant for induction.

> Several lines of evidence are consistent with normal, physiological neural induction of ectoderm by the mesodermal organizer mediated by several distinct soluble secreted proteins. The three most likely candidates are follistatin, chordin, and noggin.

Each of the three candidates not only induces neural tissue in culture experiments of ectoderm, but each is expressed in organizer tissue at the appropriate developmental time, as detected by in situ hybridization of the messenger RNA (mRNA) for the protein. In addition, when any of these molecules is expressed in isolated ectodermal cells, the formation of epidermis is inhibited and neural phenotypic properties are formed. TGF-β-like molecules induce embryonic cells to develop a mesodermal nature and thus inhibit neural formation. Mesodermal tendencies are probably driven by the TGF-β family members known as bone morphogenetic proteins (BMPs). All three putative neural inducer molecules competitively inhibit this pathway.

Disruption of the genes encoding these proteins, by homologous recombination experiments, is also useful in resolving this issue. For instance, the follistatin knockout mouse appears to be born with a relatively normal nervous system. Thus, follistatin alone is not essential for neural induction. Perhaps the other two molecules provide functional redundancy. Additional studies in which all three genes are simultaneously blocked are necessary to determine this. Finally, follistatin, noggin, and chordin induce neural tissue that is, at least in some ways, deficient in the characteristics found in neural tissue induced by contact with true organizer tissue. Based on observations such as these, there is still reasonable doubt regarding the true molecular nature of Spemann's organizer.

CELLULAR DIFFERENTIATION

Following the phenomenon of neural induction, neuronal differentiation, an equally complex developmental program, begins.

> *Cellular differentiation* is the stereotypic acquisition of the cellular and biochemical attributes of an overtly specialized cell type.

Although neurons share a number of common attributes, the wide diversity of neuronal cell types (see Chapter 1), the diversity of the cellular interactions, and the many functions of neurons engender additional intricacies for neuronal differentiation. Rather than attempting to demonstrate this in an inclusive way, this section of the chapter describes the differentiation of a large subpopulation of neural cells from the neural crest. The general features of a progressive alteration of the properties of these cells as a consequence of molecular signal transduction can be applied to other cell types of the developing nervous system.

Cell Fate

The union of sperm and oocyte and the earliest cell divisions produce totipotent cells.

> *Totipotent cells* can give rise to all of the types of cells of the organism.

The potential of these early cells is total. As development proceeds, the *prospective potency* (all possible developmental fates) of the cells is progressively more restricted. At later stages of development, this refinement of cell fate gives rise to pluripotent cells.

Pluripotent cells can generate many different cells, but not all types of cells.

The irreversible fixation of cells in a particular developmental path is known as *determination*. For example, by the end of gastrulation, the major portions of the nervous system have been determined. The *prospective significance* of cells in a specific region of the embryo is the fate of those cells if left undisturbed by curious scientists during normal development. Prospective significance has been determined by observing the migration of vital dyes and other tracers introduced into embryonic cells early in development.

Neural Crest Cell Diversity

The prospective potency of neural crest cells is particularly diverse. Neural crest cells give rise to the neurons and Schwann cells of the peripheral nervous system, the enteric nervous system of the gastrointestinal tract, the pigmented melanocytes of the skin, and in the head region, even some bony portions of the skull known as branchial or visceral arches. One hypothesis to explain the fate-determining mechanism of these multipotent cells relies on cellular environmental cues. The cell may be directed to differentiate along a specific pathway of determination based simply on where the cell is located in the body. This hypothesis is consistent with transplantation experiments similar to those previously described for Spemann's organizer. The developmental fate of crest cells is also clearly dependent on the migratory route through which the cells move toward their final destination in the body.

There are three major migratory routes for neural crest cells: *craniofacial, enteric,* and *trunk.*

Cells that will populate the head region travel along *craniofacial* routes. Soon after neurulation is complete, neural crest cells from the anterior neural tube (at the site of the developing brain) stream outward in a ventrolateral direction beneath the ectoderm. *Enteric* routes are taken by some of the crest cells generated in the anterior neural tube and others in the most posterior region. These cells

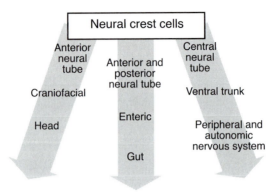

Figure 2–3
Neural crest cell migratory routes.

invade endodermal structures and take up final positions throughout the gut from the esophagus to the large bowel. In the main body of the animal, neural crest cells travel along *trunk* routes. A dorsal trunk route directs prospective melanocytes toward the overlying ectoderm. Ventral trunk routes carry the progenitors of chromaffin cells of the adrenal medulla and the neurons and Schwann cells of the peripheral nervous system including the sensory dorsal root ganglion neurons and the effector neurons of the sympathetic nervous system (Figure 2–3).

When neural crest cells move out along the ventral trunk route and reach the base of the neural tube, the cells become committed to a sympathoadrenal progenitor fate (Figure 2–4). These same cells, if analyzed earlier in development before

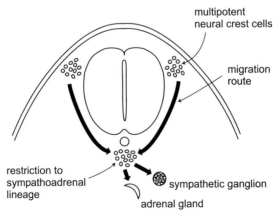

Figure 2–4
The migration route of neural crest cells restricts differentiation to sympathetic neurons or adrenal chromaffin cells. See text for details.

moving to this location, are capable of the full multipotent range. But now, at this point, these cells will develop into sympathetic neurons, adrenal chromaffin cells, or a third minor cell type, the small intensely fluorescent (SIF) cell. The final specification of these progenitor cells appears to be controlled by diffusible signals in the extracellular space. Among other polypeptide growth factors, nerve growth factor (NGF) directs these progenitor cells toward the phenotype of sympathetic neurons. On the other hand, cells that encounter high concentrations of glucocorticoids (present in the adrenal cortex) assume the properties of adrenal chromaffin cells.

Molecular Signal Transduction

> *Molecular signal transduction* is the process by which specific signals at the cell membrane result in the determination of neural cell fate.

The identification of these specific signals remains a challenge. In those cases in which putative extracellular molecules have been isolated, the challenge has shifted to understanding the intracellular events responsible for the cellular response. Figure 2–5 illustrates only a few of the potential interacting intracellular signaling cascades that are set in motion on ligand binding to cell surface receptors. Within minutes or less after ligand binding, many different enzyme systems are activated. Some receptors are themselves kinases or serve as scaffolds for the binding of intracellular proteins that possess enzymatic activities. It is impossible to include all of the intracellular targets of the activated enzymes depicted, in part because the figure would be too crowded, but primarily because not all of the targets are known! At the crossroads of several of these signal-transduction pathways is the family of kinases referred to as extracellular signal-regulated kinases (ERKs). This so-called signal-transduction cassette has downstream targets that have functions throughout the cell (at membranes, in the cytoplasm, or associated with the cytoskeleton or the nucleus). Because this signal-transduction pathway is involved in responses as diverse as cell proliferation and cell differentiation, it is not surprising that the pathway is subject to many potential upstream regulatory signals and acts on numerous downstream cellular targets.

The large number of potential combinations of signal interactions and subsequent effects is intimidating to contemplate. Discerning the biological and chemical rules that govern signal transduction is one of the major frontiers in cell biology today. In the face of this daunting complexity, it is shortsighted to conclude there is a simple explanation for what occurs inside a cell. A more constructive view of the field concedes that the generation of a biological machine as complex as the vertebrate nervous system is likely to require numerous checks and balances to complete the developmental program successfully and reproducibly.

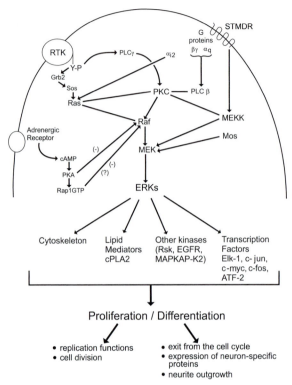

Figure 2–5

Potential signal-transduction cascades involved in neuronal development. Receptors (RTK, receptor tyrosine kinases; STMDR, seven transmembrane domain receptors, and others not shown) activate enzymes (PLC$_\gamma$, PLC$_\beta$, specific phospholipases; PKC, protein kinase C; PKA, protein kinase A; MEK, MAP/ERK kinase; MEKK, MEK kinase; ERK, extracellular signal-regulated kinase) or promote the formation of protein–protein complexes that send signals through the cytoplasm to the cytoskeleton or the nucleus.

One principle of signal transduction is that the type of receptors expressed on the cell surface is a primary determinant of the types of signals and the spectrum of responses that a particular cell acquires. Thus, receptor expression helps to shape the developmental fate of cells.

Some of the intracellular targets that are cell type–specific may also confer quite different properties on cells. An instructive example is the finding that two very closely related kinases, Raf-1 and Raf-B, are associated with opposing effects: Raf-1 activity is associated with cell proliferation and Raf-B activity can stimulate neuronal differentiation. As more is learned about signal-transduction cascades and intracellular signaling targets, it can be envisioned that pharmaceutical and biotechnological interventions will alleviate or even prevent many developmental processes of disease.

In summary, the diversity of signal-transduction events responsible for neuronal development should rightfully be viewed in the context of the wide diversity of cell types generated in the brain. What can be responsible for the genesis of a cerebellar granule neuron rather than a Betz cell from layer V in the primary motor cortex? The rules of signal transduction are no doubt the key to understanding the differences and the similarities. Signal transduction is a guidepost for development. Scientists are fond of pointing out that when one of these rules is discovered in a species, it turns out to be equally applicable in other species, including humans.

CELL MIGRATION

Another common principle of neuronal development is cell migration.

> *Cell migration* is the migration of nascent nerve cells, like those of the neural crest, from their birthplace to their final location.

Virtually all neural cells in the developing brain migrate from a site of origin near the cerebral ventricles to sites at varying distances from the ventricular lumen. These *ventricular zones* are the centers for cell proliferation within the pseudostratified neuroepithelium of the neural tube. Later in the period of cortical neurogenesis, secondary germinal centers form in areas overlying the ventricular zone. This *subventricular zone* provides a secondary wave of neurogenesis for the extremely large number of cells that comprise the cerebral and cerebellar cortices. The subventricular zones in humans are capable of neurogenesis for at least two years after birth. The final cell division that gives rise to a postmitotic neuron (i.e., no longer capable of dividing) is termed the *neuronal birthday.*

> After precursor proliferation is complete, postmitotic neurons migrate away from the germinal centers to form the different laminae of the nervous system.

Neurons that are "born" first take up final residence close to the ventricular zone. Later generations of neurons migrate further and inhabit more distant brain layers. There are two main categories of neuronal migration: (1) neurons that are attracted to move preferentially along the surfaces of other neurons and (2) neurons that migrate along routes determined by radial glia or by adhesive molecules in the extracellular matrix. Radial glial cells are among the first cells to differentiate. These cells can provide physical "guides" enabling neurons to move from the proliferative zones toward the surface of the brain. Research on radial glial guides indicates that the glial processes extending radially away from the proliferative areas toward the surface of the brain serve a permissive rather than a specifically instructive role. Neurons from many different brain regions can migrate equally well on the same glial fibers. As described previously for neural crest cells, differentiation is not normally completed until the cells establish permanent residence.

The molecular mechanisms involved in migration are not yet clear.

> Receptors on the surface of migrating cells are responsible for sensing location and regulating motile behavior.

One such neuronal receptor is *astrotactin,* found on granule neurons of the cerebellum. The ligands that activate these receptors may be diffusible molecules or may be found on the surface of other cells. The *Slit* family of proteins, originally identified in the fruit fly, appears to serve as one form of diffusible cue. In addition, all cells secrete proteins that comprise a heterogeneous mixture of insoluble material referred to as *extracellular matrix.* Cell type–specific secretions can generate locally variable compositions of the extracellular matrix that interact with the receptors of migrating cells. This variety of chemically active, regionally specific, insoluble cues is another means by which migrating neurons receive orders either to stop migrating or to continue migrating to a more appropriate final destination.

Additional research is required to elucidate the specific intracellular events that are set in motion by the receptors of migrating neuronal precursors. Interestingly, however, it appears that the functional response produced by ligand binding to cell surface receptors can function in two ways. First, receptor engagement may activate cell adhesion and neuronal precursor migration along a defined route. Alternatively, some receptors may carry out *chemorepellent* functions (as in the case of *Slit*) to guide the migration by preventing the neuronal precursor from moving in the direction of high concentrations of the ligand.

PROCESS OUTGROWTH

Growth Cones

> The connectivity between neurons in the brain requires the generation of long, thin processes that carry outgoing information (*axons*) and shorter, more tapered processes that receive information (*dendrites*).

The function of Sherrington's enchanted loom is critically dependent on the proper outgrowth of these processes from the nerve cell body.

> The most important structural feature of the growing axons and dendrites is the *growth cone,* which is a specialized structure at the distal tip of processes.

The growth cone (Figure 2–6) was originally described in fixed histological sections of animal embryos by the father of developmental neurobiology, Ramon y Cajal. Ross Harrison, who invented modern tissue culture during his pioneering studies of neuronal development, first observed growth cones in the living state. With increased refinements of his techniques, it is now widely appreciated that growth cones are among the most dynamic biological structures known, changing dramatically over a time scale of minutes.

The most active area of the growth cone is the distal membrane called the *lamellipodium,* a fine veil-like structure that explores the surrounding environment in all three dimensions. Thin, finger-like projections, called *filopodia,* are composed of bundles of actin filaments extending from the thick, organelle-rich central domain of the growth cone. Focal swellings along the shaft of the growing process have been called *varicosities.* The varicosity may contribute membrane and other components to the end of the shaft where growth occurs. The specialized growth cone also coordinates navigation through the developing brain tissue. Regulation of growth and navigation is mediated by instruc-

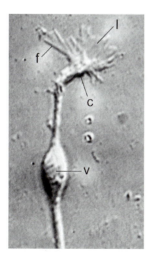

Figure 2–6
Neuronal growth cone in cell culture.
l, lamellipodium; f, filopodium; c, organelle-rich central domain of the growth cone; v, varicosity.

tional ligands that serve either as chemoattractants or as cues that repel the advancing growth cone.

As in migration of neurons, growth cones are guided by extracellular markers and diffusible molecules.

Extracellular matrix contains laminin and fibronectin. Growth cones have integrin receptors that bind to laminin and fibronectin. This binding activates second messenger cascades that promote neurite outgrowth. There are also cadherins, found in both the growth cones and target cells, which promote outgrowth. In addition, there is a family of cell adhesion molecules (CAMs) that promotes cell–cell interactions. There are nerve cell adhesion molecules (N-CAMs) that foster interactions between axons to form nerve fiber bundles, and there are nerve glial cell adhesion molecules (Ng-CAMs) that promote axon outgrowth along glial cells. Perturbation of Ng-CAM function can lead to motor neuron diseases in neonates.

Axon Targeting

Roger Sperry sought to account for the specificity of axon growth in the nervous system with his *chemoaffinity hypothesis*. This experimental model, worked out in the retinotectal system of animals (see Chapter 11), proposes that

axon–target connections are governed by chemical labels that identify each axon and target cell.

Although Sperry did not specifically identify any of the recognition molecules involved in generating the final "wiring diagram" of the nervous system, his hypothesis spawned countless experiments to discover such molecules. Nerve growth factor (NGF), the first neurotrophic substance to be discovered, was seized on as validation of Sperry's hypothesis.

Neurotrophism refers to a nourishing or survival-promoting function between target cells and the innervating neurons.

Rita Levi-Montalcini, who like Sperry won the Nobel Prize, demonstrated that NGF promotes axon outgrowth from sympathetic and sensory neurons.

Target tissues innervated by these neurons produce significant quantities of NGF mRNA and protein at the appropriate time of development. Finally, experiments in cell culture dramatically illustrated how a moving source of soluble NGF can reorient the path of axon growth over a time course of less than 2 hours. These latter studies, performed in cell culture, indicate that

nerve growth factor is also a *neurotropic* substance, an agent that orients or guides the growing process toward the target.

NGF was cloned in 1983. With the ascendancy of recombinant genetic technology, homologous genes were isolated in rapid succession. Table 2–2 illustrates the members of the expanded neurotrophin family. Brain-derived neurotrophic factor (BDNF) and neurotrophin 3 (NT3) share ~ 50% structural conservation with NGF.

Each neurotrophin can bind to at least two cell surface receptors. All bind to the relatively low-affinity site, p75, and a second high-affinity Trk receptor. NGF binds to TrkA, BDNF and NT4/5 bind to TrkB, and NT3 binds to TrkC.

NT3 also exhibits weaker binding interactions with TrkA and TrkB. All neurotrophins promote neurite outgrowth from dorsal root ganglion (DRG) neurons

Table 2–2 NEUROTROPHINS, PROCESS OUTGROWTH, AND RECEPTORS[a,b]								
Neurotrophin	DRG	SCG	Ciliary	Nodose	TrkA	TrkB	TrkC	p75
NGF	++	++	–	–	√			√
BDNF	++	–	–	+		√		√
NT3	++	±	–	++	•	•	√	√
NT4/5	++	–/±	?	±/–		√		√
NT6[c]						√		
NT7[d]						√		

[a]–, No neurite outgrowth; ±, little or no neurite outgrowth; +, neurite outgrowth; ++, robust neurite outgrowth; ?, not tested; √, binds well; •, binds weakly.
[b]DRG, dorsal root ganglion; SCG, superior cervical ganglion; NGF, nerve growth factor; BDNF, brain-derived neurotrophic factor; NT, neurotrophin.
[c]In teleost fish (biological actions similar to NGF).
[d]Presently found only in zebra fish.

in culture, but only NGF produces a significant response from postnatal sympathetic superior cervical ganglion (SCG) neurons, and NT3 is the most efficient neurotrophin for promoting neurite outgrowth from parasympathetic nodose ganglion neurons. Thus, neurotrophin signaling specificity is imposed by cell type–specific expression of neurotrophin receptors. The potential diversity of neuronal responsiveness in the developing brain is emphasized further by the large number of other families of soluble neurite-promoting substances, including *neurturins, netrins, ephrins, semaphorins,* other members of the *TGF-β family,* and an ever-expanding list of *cytokines.* Comparatively speaking, each of these ligands associates with receptor systems that exhibit equally complex ligand-binding interactions. For example, semaphorins are a group of molecules that can regulate neurite outgrowth. They selectively repel some neurons, while promoting outgrowth from others. In another example, netrins promote growth of commissural axons but inhibit the growth of other nerve fibers. Thus, they serve as gatekeepers of decussating nerve fibers.

Trophic factors may also be released by neurons and affect their target cells. One particularly well-studied example is agrin, which is released by motor neurons. Agrin promotes the aggregation of acetylcholine receptors at the postsynaptic region of muscle fibers. Animals with agrin knockouts have severely reduced numbers of neuromuscular junctions.

Based on the previous discussion, it may appear that the broad spectrum of recognition molecules and receptors could possibly account for the amazing specificity envisioned by Sperry. However, the definitive explanation of how axons are guided to specific target sites is more likely to be determined by several sequential mechanisms rather than simple one-to-one chemical affinities. In addition to selective soluble guidance cues, insoluble extracellular matrix molecules and even anatomical landmarks can serve to promote neurite outgrowth. Recognition of the proper target may rely on a different set of cues. The electrical activity patterns of individual neurons and competition among many chemical signals are also major influences on the establishment of proper neuronal connections. Completion of the multifactorial phenomenon of process outgrowth is the culmination of a critical developmental landmark. Simultaneous with the conclusion of process outgrowth is the initiation of the next principal stage of neuronal development, synaptogenesis.

SYNAPTOGENESIS AND PROGRAMMED CELL DEATH

Synapse Formation

Neuronal differentiation continues throughout the principal stages of the development of the nervous system (see Table 2–1). The earliest stages of induction and the neuronal birthday confer phenotypic and functional properties such as exit from the cell cycle and the synthesis of neuron-specific proteins. The most important functional property of neurons is the capacity for rapid long-range communication. The development of this function depends on the generation of the morphological structure of the communicating junction between the innervating nerve cell and target, the *synapse*.

Synaptogenesis is the formation of synapses.

The types of synapses formed in the nervous system are as diverse as the types of neurons generated during development. The establishment of each type involves an exchange of signals that leads to further functional differentiation of both the innervating neuron and its target. There are many sources of these signals. At the neuromuscular junction, a well-studied synapse, there is a very specialized extracellular matrix known as the synaptic *basal lamina*. Protein molecules in this structure provide a distinctive and restricted location on the muscle cell for synapse formation. Neurotransmitters and other biochemicals secreted by the presynaptic neuron contribute to synapse formation by modifying the properties of the postsynaptic cell. Hormones, such as the sex steroids estrogen and testosterone, play important, though poorly understood, roles in conferring gender-specific differences in CNS organization and behavior. Target-derived signals are critically necessary for proper synapse formation: they maintain the synapse and ensure the survival of the presynaptic neuron.

Developmental Cell Death

Stereotyped cell death in both the central and peripheral nervous systems has long been known to result in the loss of 50% or more of all the neurons born in a given brain region. This naturally occurring *programmed cell death* (PCD) begins at developmental stages immediately prior to the onset of synaptogenesis (Figure 2–7).

Neuron survival that occurs as a function of synapse formation has resulted in the formulation of the *neurotrophic hypothesis.*

One of the key findings that led to the neurotrophic hypothesis is that experimental manipulation of postsynaptic target size has a great influence on the number of neurons that survive after the developmental onset of PCD. Surgical removal of increasing amounts of the target, whether a peripheral wing bud or a CNS nucleus, leads to progressively greater losses in the number of presynaptic innervating neurons. Complementary evidence for a neurotrophic function of the

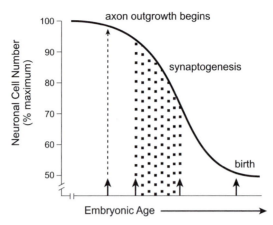

Figure 2–7
Synaptogenesis coincides temporally with programmed cell death in the developing nervous system.

synaptic connection comes from studies that increase target size, either by transplantation or other means. These experiments demonstrate that greater than normal target tissue size can induce survival in 50% to 70% of the neurons that would normally have died during development.

The neurotrophic hypothesis provides several teleological explanations for the phenomenon of embryonic PCD and the natural course of developmental events.

1. The generation of excess neurons ensures that all healthy target cells will be innervated. PCD also provides a tightly regulated mechanism for efficiently matching effector cell populations to target sizes.
2. Growth cone migration to inappropriate sites in the nervous system should be effectively eliminated.
3. A population of excess neurons may have been an evolutionarily favorable adaptation for higher animals. The establishment of more complex neuroanatomical pathways in animal brains may have required surplus neurons with which to expand the possible interconnections.

Figure 2–8 schematically illustrates the neurotrophic hypothesis. A presynaptic population of neurons with axons racing toward their target tissue (Figure 2–8A) competes for a finite number of synaptic sites. After the synapse is established, neurotrophic substances, such as NGF, can be taken up by the neuronal ending and transported back to the nerve cell body by *retrograde axonal flow.* Because the quantity of the trophic substances is limited, only a select fraction of the neurons survives. The unsuccessful embryonic neurons will die in a characteristically quiet manner typical of PCD (Figure 2–8B), with no associated inflammation or injury response. As with all of the other principal stages of neu-

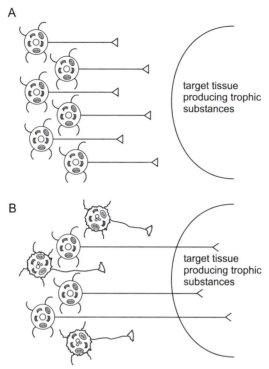

Figure 2–8
The neurotrophic hypothesis. Approximately 50% of the initial neuronal population (**A**) will survive after synaptogenesis (**B**) due to a limited supply of neurotrophic substances in the target tissue.

ronal development discussed in this chapter, there are specific molecular and intracellular biochemical signals important for survival and further differentiation that are triggered by trophic factor interaction with neuronal receptors. Perhaps even more important is the default signaling pathway, which is initiated in the absence of trophic signaling. In this case, a different cascade of molecular and biochemical events is set in motion for the time-dependent, silent execution of the neuron. There is some provocative and interesting recent evidence that implicates the p75 NGF receptor in the activation of cell death programs.

SYNAPTIC REMODELING
AND STRUCTURAL ALTERATIONS

The formation of synapses is not the conclusion of neuronal development. Synapses are initially produced in excess of what is necessary in the adult animal. Mechanisms for synaptic elimination are dependent on the pattern and strength of presynaptic neuronal activity. The refinement of synaptic connections and the capacity of the nervous system to eliminate and recreate synapses well into adulthood are properties shared by many highly evolved species, particularly *Homo sapiens.*

Synaptic remodeling and alterations of synapses in the nervous system occur during critical periods in neuronal development.

Throughout the life of higher animals, behavioral adjustments such as learning and memory require this sort of reorganization of structural connections between neurons. Injury to the nerves and tracts of the nervous system because of disease or trauma also promotes cellular and biochemical adjustments that mount a regenerative response to reestablish damaged areas.

Critical Periods

Critical periods are discrete times of neuronal development during which newly forming synaptic connections require appropriate activity or input from the environment for normal developmental maturation and function.

These critical periods operate in a wide variety of events ranging from the acquisition of specific physiological responses in the visual system to the complex behavioral adaptations of young animals. The development of binocular vision in mammals, essential for depth perception, occurs during a critical period, as does the learning of a species-specific birdsong by young songbirds, which takes place in early postnatal life. These developmental landmarks involve specific centers in the brain in which both electrical activity and chemical signaling play roles in establishing and maintaining these responses through synaptic connections.

In the case of birdsong, for example, the establishment of sexually dimorphic areas of the CNS depends on exposure of the songbird to the song of an adult male bird of the same species and the influence of sex steroids, both of which are crucial during postnatal critical periods. Although female birds vocalize, only young male birds are capable of learning the species-specific song from adult male birds during the critical period. Estrogen is important for organizing the areas of the CNS involved in birdsong. As the androgen, testosterone, rises abruptly during sexual maturation, the critical period for learning birdsong closes and the song pattern produced is stabilized.

Another famous example of a complex behavior triggered during a critical period is *imprinting*. Konrad Lorenz, the world-renowned ethologist, first demonstrated the phenomenal regard that a newborn animal exhibits for the first sizable moving object that it encounters early in life. The animal comes to regard this object as representative of its species. There is a unique bonding between this object, usually the animal's parent, and the neonate. In some birds this critical period can be as short as several hours immediately after birth. Lorenz dramatically demonstrated this principle many times by allowing the newborn to imprint on lifeless, moving objects, or even himself, as substitutes for the natural parent.

These examples and the principles observed in the research on critical periods in animals are directly applicable to complex human developmental programs, such as the acquisition of language skills.

Injury and Regeneration in the Nervous System

The study of the cellular and molecular mechanisms involved in normal neuronal development has implications for studies in human biology and treatment of disease at all ages.

A complete understanding of the elements involved in promoting process outgrowth during development can provide useful insights into the facilitation of neuronal regeneration following tissue damage caused by injury or disease.

Whereas peripheral nerves that are damaged are capable of complete regeneration with full functional recovery, the CNS when damaged is not. *Axotomy,* the interruption of neural connections, leads to the up-regulation of specific growth-associated genes in neurons of both the PNS and the CNS. In the PNS, however, neurotrophic factors and extracellular matrix molecules that combine to promote growth in nerve bundles are much more prevalent than in the nerve tracts of the CNS. In the CNS of the adult, there are two additional major impediments to axon regeneration: (1) an increased tendency for glial scarring to form around cut axonal endings making regeneration through the scar tissue difficult; and (2) a large number of potent inhibitors of neurite growth. Therapies for spinal cord and brain injuries will rely on a better understanding of the growth-promoting influences that operate during development as well as the molecules that inhibit growth, particularly with regard to the intracellular response triggered by these molecules.

Neurodegenerative Diseases

An exciting, though formidable frontier for additional research is the area of neurodegenerative diseases. Many neurological conditions, including Alzheimer disease, Parkinson disease, and amyotrophic lateral sclerosis (Lou Gehrig's disease), share the common attribute of an inexplicable death of nerve cells in discrete areas of the brain. These illnesses strike adult men and women.

> One current attractive hypothesis to account for nerve cell loss in neurodegenerative diseases is the inappropriate activation of specific PCD signals that normally operate only during early brain development.

For unknown etiological reasons, these programs may be activated later in life in a pathological context. Because PCD is a multistep signaling cascade, as previously discussed, this hypothesis offers the potential for therapeutic interventions that would interrupt or reverse the program. Based on this possibility, the field of neuronal PCD has expanded to enormous proportions in a search for the critical intracellular signaling steps that commit the neuron to its silent suicide.

Potential approaches to treat neurodegenerative diseases include pharmacological and/or gene therapies. Drugs that selectively affect intracellular signal transduction pathways may be useful in enhancing intracellular survival signals or dampening the pathological activation of cell death. There are also a number of genes that when activated provide neuroprotective actions by scavenging cell-damaging oxygen free radicals or have other beneficial functions. The ultimate usefulness of any of these options for the treatment of disease depends on the specificity of the cellular and molecular actions of the intervention. Thus, once again, a complete description of the functions of the intracellular signal-transduction elements involved is necessary for the success of this endeavor. This is one of the many exciting research challenges facing developmental neurobiologists.

· C H A P T E R · 3 ·

NEURONAL SIGNALING

·

Malcolm Slaughter

Membrane Potentials

Action Potentials

Cable Properties

Synaptic Potentials

Presynaptic Modulation of Transmitter Release

Postsynaptic Plasticity

•   •   •   •   •   •   •   •   •   •   •   •

MEMBRANE POTENTIALS

Although most cells in the body maintain a potential of about -70 mV, in excitable cells such as nerve and muscle cells this potential can vary. This regulation can result in action potentials, muscle contraction, or neurotransmitter release. The controlled regulation of membrane potential allows neurons to integrate complex information. For these reasons neuroscience has explored the mechanisms that control membrane potential.

Formation of the Membrane Potential

Neurons, like most other cells in the body, contain a slight excess of negative charge. This means that the voltages inside cells are more negative, usually by about 70 mV, than the extracellular space.

> Neurons can rapidly change their voltage (electrical potential) by changing the charges that enter or leave the cell (Figure 3–1). Charge is carried by ions: *anions* (Cl^-) and *cations* (Na^+, K^+, and Ca^{2+}).

The membrane potential of a cell depends on the permeability and concentration gradient of ions across the membrane. If an ion cannot cross the membrane (low permeability), it cannot change the neuron's membrane potential. If an ion is permeable, the effect on membrane potential will depend on the charge of the ion and the way in which it will move.

> The direction of movement depends on two parameters: the *electrical gradient* and the *concentration gradient*.

For each ion these two gradients are related by the Nernst equation:

$$E = (58/n) \times \log([\text{cation outside}]/[\text{cation inside}])$$

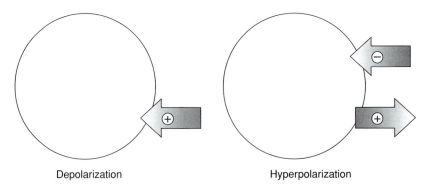

Depolarization   Hyperpolarization

Figure 3–1
Ion movement and membrane voltage. Neurons are depolarized by the entrance of positive ions (sodium or calcium). Neurons are hyperpolarized by the entrance of negative ions (chloride) or the exit of positive ions (potassium).

where E is the equilibrium (or reversal) potential measured in millivolts, n is the valence of the ion, and the terms in brackets denote concentration. For example, if the concentration of sodium ion (Na^+, an ion with one positive charge, $n = +1$) is 10 times higher outside the cell than inside the cell, the above equation indicates that a cell permeable to sodium and with these relative concentrations of sodium inside and outside the cell will have the following potential:

$$E = (58/1) \times \log([10]/[1]) = +58 \text{ mV}$$

If chloride (Cl^-, $n = -1$) were 10 times higher outside the cell than inside the cell, the cell would have the following potential:

$$E = (58/-1) \times \log([10]/[1]) = (-58) \times 1 = -58 \text{ mV}$$

The equilibrium potentials for Ca^{2+}, Na^+, Cl^-, and K^+ are approximately +100 mV, +60 mV, −75 mV (variable), and −90 mV, respectively.

So far we have discussed the effect of a single ion crossing the cell membrane. In reality, the potential of a cell depends on the *collective equilibrium potentials and permeabilities* (P) of all the ions, as described by the Goldman equation:

$$E = 58 \log \left(\frac{P_{Na}[Na]_o + P_K[K]_o + P_{Cl}[Cl]_i}{P_{Na}[Na]_i + P_K[K]_i + P_{Cl}[Cl]_o} \right)$$

This is similar to the Nernst equation, except that the permeabilities (P) of each ion are considered. Essentially, the final membrane potential depends on the Nernst potential for each ion and the relative permeabilities of the ions.

The *resting potential* of neurons is dominated by a potassium conductance and is about −70 mV (note that if it were exclusively dependent on potassium, then the resting potential would be −90 mV).

Inhibitory (hyperpolarizing) potentials are the result of an increase in potassium or chloride permeability. *Excitatory* (depolarizing) potentials are produced by an increase in sodium or calcium permeability.

Pumps

The electrical potential across the cell membrane depends on unequal concentrations of ions inside and outside the cell.

For most cells, the concentration of potassium is much higher inside the cell (C_{out} = 5 mM and C_{in} = 150 mM), and the concentration of sodium is much higher outside the cell (Figure 3–2). The concentration gradients are thermodynamically unfavorable, meaning that energy is required to establish and to maintain these gradients. The gradients are formed by pumps, which use the energy from adenosine triphosphate (ATP) to move (concentrate) ions inside or outside the cell.

The pumps are often referred to as adenosine triphosphatases (ATPases), such as the *Na^+/K^+-ATPase,* which is a protein in the membrane that pumps three sodium ions out of the cell for every two potassium ions pumped in (Figure 3–2).

Note that this produces a net outward movement of one positive charge, and therefore this is an electrogenic pump that hyperpolarizes the cell. The Na^+/K^+-ATPase, commonly called the *sodium pump,* can be blocked by ouabain, resulting in the loss of the Na^+ and K^+ concentration gradients, reduction in membrane potential, and cell death. Na^+/K^+-ATPase is a single protein that crosses the membrane 10 times. The protein has an internal ATP binding site, an internal phosphorylation site, an intramembrane potassium binding site, and an extracellular ouabain binding site.

Another commonly found pump is Ca^{2+}-ATPase, which pumps calcium out of the cell. The internal calcium concentrations of neurons are very low (about 100 nM in resting cells), whereas the extracellular concentration is about 2 mM. The maintenance of both this very low internal concentration and this very large concentration gradient (20,000-fold) is essential for many neuronal processes such as synaptic transmission.

There is another set of membrane proteins that uses the gradients generated by pumps to create additional concentration gradients. These are exchangers, which move one ion down its energy gradient and link this thermodynamically favorable process to the movement of another ion against its concentration gradient. For example, the Na^+/Ca^{2+} exchanger links the movement of sodium into a cell (favorable) with the movement of calcium outward. Note that the exchanger did not

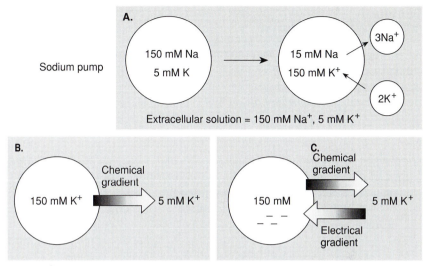

Gradient provides energy for formation of the membrane potential
and for the transport of some substances across the cell membrane

Figure 3–2
(**A**) Pumps use ATP to concentrate potassium inside the cell while keeping the
intracellular sodium concentration low. (**B**) The resting membrane potential is dictated
mainly by potassium. (**C**) Because of the chemical (concentration) gradient, potassium
exits the cell and thus makes the inside of the cell negative. Eventually, this electrical
gradient balances the concentration gradient. This forms a chemical (concentration)
gradient that favors the removal of potassium.

require an energy source such as ATP, but depends indirectly on Na^+/K^+-ATPase
to generate the potential energy of the sodium gradient.

Channels

Ions cannot pass through the lipid membrane, but pass through pores formed
by channel proteins that sit ("float") in the lipid membrane.

Channels are *selective* for particular ions. The selectivity can be for anions
or cations, or for particular ions such as sodium-selective channels or
potassium-selective channels.

Ion channel *conductance* is a measure of the ease with which ions pass
through the pore. It is the inverse of *resistance* and follows Ohm's law, $I = gV$,
where I is current, g is conductance, and V is voltage.

Relationship Between Single-Channel Currents and Membrane Potential

1. Current flow through a single channel in time has the shape of a *rectangular pulse.* Each channel acts as a conductor and a battery.
2. *Total current* flow across a membrane, which contains many identical channels, is simply the sum of the currents through single channels:

$$I_{total} = NPi$$

where I_{total} is the total cell membrane current, N is the total number of channels available in the membrane, P is the probability that a channel is open, and i is the current through a single channel.

3. The value of the *resting membrane potential* is determined by the total current and cell resistance, according to Ohm's law.

Gating

Channel proteins can change conformation so that the channel is either opened or closed to the passage of ions. This property of channels, called *gating,* is the most important mechanism for the regulation of channels.

Three parameters control gating: voltage, ligands (neurotransmitters), and mechanical forces. Channel proteins can be described by these three parameters. For example, one channel involved in producing the action potential is a sodium-selective channel (Figure 3–3), of approximately 25 picosiemen (pS) conductance that is gated by voltage (opens when the cell is depolarized). The prototypical ligand-gated channel is opened by acetylcholine, is selective for both sodium and potassium, and has a conductance of 25 pS (Figure 3–4). In the auditory system, mechanically gated channels on the cilia of hair cells are responsible for the transduction of sound to bioelectrical activity.

This main gate, which determines whether ions will pass through the channel, is called the *activation gate.* In some channels there is another gate called the *inactivation gate.*

The inactivation gate, which may also be voltage dependent, usually moves more slowly than the activation gate and mirrors the response of the activation

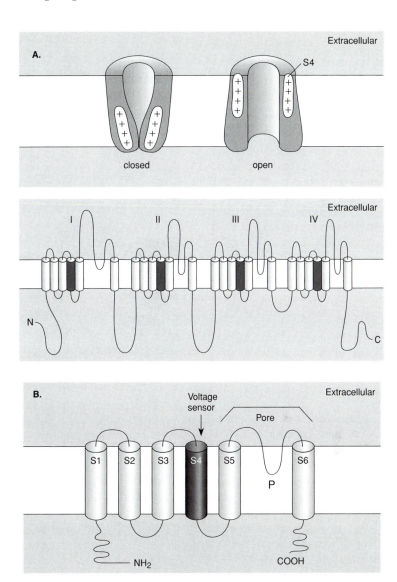

Figure 3–3
Voltage-gated channels are made of proteins that cross the membrane many times.
(**A**) (**Top**) Functional components and (**bottom**) peptide folding. The main subunit of voltage-gated sodium and calcium channels has four domains (I–IV); in each domain the protein crosses the membrane six times. The fourth crossing (S4) of each domain combines to form the voltage sensor. The loop (P-loop) between the fifth and sixth membrane crossings (S5 and S6) forms the pore of the channel. (**B**) The voltage-gated potassium channel may contain subunits equivalent to only one domain of the sodium or calcium channel.

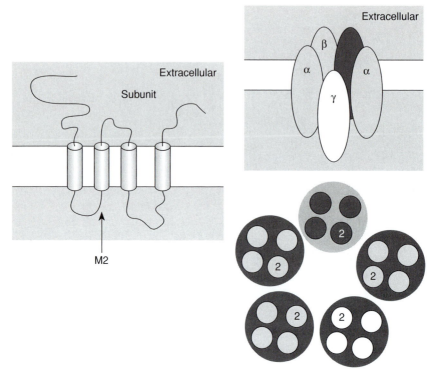

Figure 3–4
Ligand-gated channels, such as the acetylcholine, γ-aminobutyric acid, and glycine receptors, consist of five subunits. Each subunit crosses the membrane four times. The second crossing of each subunit (M2) forms the pore in the acetylcholine channel.

gate. Using the voltage-activated sodium channel as an example (Figure 3–5), under resting conditions (–70 mV), most sodium channels have their activation gate closed and their inactivation gate open. Because both gates must be open to enable ions to pass, the channel is effectively closed. Cell depolarization can open the activation gate, allowing the flow of ions, but the inactivation gate then closes, preventing further ionic flow. The sodium channel stays in this inactivated state until the cell is hyperpolarized back to –70 mV, at which point the activation gate closes and the inactivation gate opens. The net effect of the inactivation gate is to make sodium flux through the channel transient, even if the cell is depolarized for a prolonged time.

Electrical Units

Electrical units are defined as follows:

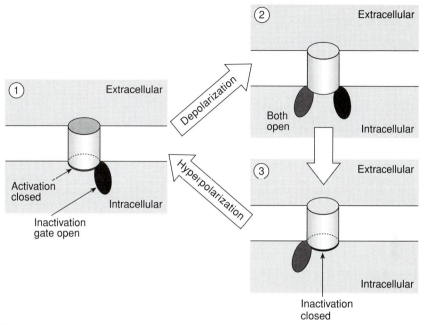

Figure 3–5

Activation and inactivation of the voltage-gated sodium channel. (1) At resting potentials (–70 mV) the activation gate is closed and the inactivation gate is open. (2) During a depolarization the activation gate opens and sodium ions can pass through the channel. (3) While the membrane is still depolarized, the inactivation gate closes, blocking the pore. The channel remains blocked until the channel returns to its original state after a hyperpolarization.

1. *Voltage* (V) is a measure of potential energy per unit charge, measured in volts (V). Biological voltages are in the range of ±100 mV.
2. *Current* (I) is a measure of the rate of flow of electric charge and is measured in amperes (A). Biological currents are in the range of picoamperes (pA, 10^{-12} A) to nanoamperes (nA, 10^{-9} A).
3. *Conductance* (g) is a measure of the ease of flow of ions and is measured in siemens (S). Its inverse is *resistance* (R), which is measured in ohms. The conductance of biological membranes is in the microsiemen (10^{-6}) to nanosiemen range.
4. *Ohm's law* relates these quantities: $V = IR$ or $I = Vg$.
5. *Capacitance* (C) is the ability to store or separate charge and is measured in farads. Membrane capacitance tends to slow the voltage response to a synaptic current. This response delay, termed a time constant, is equal to $R \times C$.

6. An *ion* is an atom or molecule bearing an electric charge, with cations being positively charged and anions being negatively charged. Some important ions in biological systems are Na^+, K^+, Ca^{2+}, Cl^-.

ACTION POTENTIALS
Voltage-Gated Channels

> Channels may be gated by changing transmembrane voltage. Most voltage-gated channels open when the cell is depolarized away from the resting potential of −70 mV.

The probability the channel will be open increases with depolarization until a maximum open probability is reached. Two channels (sodium channel and potassium channel) that combine to produce the classic action potential respond in this manner.

Properties   Voltage-gated channels possess the following properties:

1. The probability of channel *openings* depends on membrane *voltage.*
2. For most channels, open probability increases as the cell depolarizes.
3. The channel contains a *voltage sensor* that regulates the channel gate.
4. The channel may also contain voltage-sensitive *inactivation* gates.

Structure   The *calcium and sodium channels* have similar structures (Figure 3–3).

- Multiple subunits form the channel.
- There is one principal subunit (*alpha—α*) that alone can form a voltage-sensitive channel.
- The α-subunit consists of one long polypeptide containing *four domains* (I–IV).
- Each of these domains of the α-subunit crosses the membrane six times (S1–S6)
- There is a *P-loop* between S5 and S6 of the α-subunit that dips into the membrane.
- The *beta (β)-subunit* is attached to the cytoplasmic side of the α-subunit.

The *potassium channel* has the following structures:

- The α-subunit has a single domain containing S1–S6.

- It probably forms *tetramers,* which may be equivalent to the four domains of sodium and calcium channel α-subunits.

Structure–Function

- The *S4* region of the α-subunit contains positively charged amino acids that act as a voltage sensor.
- The *P-loop* of the α-subunit forms the pore and determines ion selectivity.
- The *cytoplasmic loop* between domains III and IV of the sodium channel α-subunit mediates inactivation.
- The β-subunit shifts the voltage sensitivity. In calcium channels, the β-subunit enhances the current as much as 10-fold.

For many voltage-gated channels the amino acid sequence is known, and for some the three-dimensional structure has been discerned. Voltage-gated channels are commonly formed by one long protein (α-subunit) that consists of four very similar domains. Within each domain the protein traverses the membrane six times (Figure 3–3A), and the fourth transmembrane segment (S4) contains several charged amino acids.

> When the cell's voltage changes, these charged amino acids move, and this movement causes the gate to open or close.

Another part of the domain is a short loop that folds into the membrane. This loop (called the *P-loop* or *H5*), which is between the fifth and sixth transmembrane domains, is important in forming the actual channel through which ions travel. Altering this loop can change the selectivity or the conductance of the channel. In some channels inactivation is produced by a *cytoplasmic loop* of the α-subunit, which is thought to move into the channel mouth and clog the path. The voltage-gated channel is composed not only of this long protein, called the α-subunit, but also of several ancillary subunits (β, γ, etc.) that are attached to the main α-subunit and subtly alter the channel's properties. For example, the β-subunit of some calcium channels greatly increases the current-carrying capacity of the channel.

This general description is appropriate for voltage-activated sodium and calcium channels. Voltage-sensitive potassium channels are slightly different and show more diversity. For example, some potassium channels consist of a much shorter protein that is equivalent to a single domain of the sodium or calcium channel, but four of these proteins band together to make the equivalent of the four domains.

Graded Potentials and Action Potentials

Neurons control membrane potential by formation of either a graded potential or an action potential (Figure 3–6).

> *Graded potentials* can be either negative or positive changes in voltage, and they can be of variable amplitude.

They are often slow changes in potential, they do not depend on voltage-gated channels, and their propagation along a nerve is controlled by the cable properties of the cell (see below).

> In contrast, *action potentials* are only depolarizations, and they arise from graded potentials that cause the stimulation of voltage-gated channels.

Action potentials have two unique properties: they have a threshold (initiated when a cell is depolarized to a specific voltage) and they have a fixed amplitude (called the all-or-none property) (Figure 3–7). Unlike graded potentials, action potentials can propagate unattenuated for long distances. This nondecremental con-

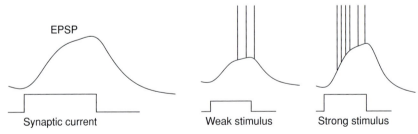

Graded potentials:
1. Variable amplitude
2. Positive or negative (EPSP or IPSP)
3. Slow

Action potentials:
1. All-or-none
2. Spike frequency $\propto$ EPSP amplitude
3. Fast, stereotyped response
4. Threshold for activation

EPSP

Synaptic current   Weak stimulus   Strong stimulus

Figure 3–6
Electrical signals in neurons. Graded potentials are slow voltage changes. The size of the voltage is proportional to the size of the stimulus (synaptic current). Graded potentials that reach a threshold voltage produce spikes. The frequency of spiking is proportional to the amplitude of the graded potential depolarization.

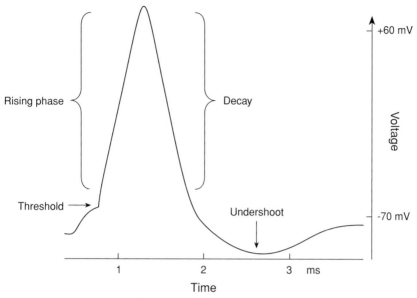

Figure 3–7
An action potential is a stereotyped response of fixed amplitude and shape. A threshold voltage change is required to initiate a spike. The rising phase is the result of sodium channel activation and the decay phase the result of potassium channel activation and sodium channel inactivation. The undershoot is the result of prolonged potassium channel activation.

duction occurs because a spike, once generated, activates the formation of a spike in the adjacent membrane segment. This is similar to a lit fuse, with every region igniting the adjacent region. An action potential can also propagate faster than a graded potential. This is most evident in myelinated nerve fibers because the action potential hops from one node of Ranvier to another, a process called *saltatory conduction*. Action potentials are initiated by graded potentials that reach the threshold voltage. A larger graded potential does not produce a larger action potential (remember the all-or-none principle), but it does produce more spikes per unit time.

Channels that Produce the Action Potential

Consider the events that lead to the classic action potential (Figure 3–7).

The first event is a depolarization that reaches threshold (usually -50 to -40 mV).

At threshold a large number of voltage-gated sodium channels open and sodium rushes into the cell. This huge influx of sodium overwhelms the influence of all other channels so that the neuron is depolarized to the sodium equilibrium potential of +60 mV (this can be illustrated by the Goldman equation when P_{Na} far exceeds the P value for all other ions).

> The depolarization that opens the sodium channel initiates two other events that terminate the action potential: the stimulation of the sodium inactivation gate, which causes the closing of sodium channels, and the activation of a voltage-gated potassium channel, which allows potassium efflux from the cell and thereby hyperpolarizes the neuron.

Both of these events are slower than the sodium channel activation gate, so a full depolarization occurs before the repolarization phase takes place.

Let us return to the two gates on the sodium channel, the activation gate and the inactivation gate (Figure 3–5). If a neuron is at rest, at −70 mV, the activation gate is closed, but the inactivation gate is open. When the neuron is depolarized, the activation gate opens and sodium ions can now flow through the channel and into the cell. But the same depolarization soon closes the inactivation gate, closing the channel again (even though the activation gate is open!). Thus the channel conducts ions for only the brief period of time (1–2 msec) in which both gates are open. The channel remains in this nonconducting, inactivated state until the cell is hyperpolarized. Then the inactivation gate opens, but the activation gate closes. So again the channel does not conduct; it now returns to its original state and is available for activation.

Sodium channel inactivation has another function. As the action potential progresses down a nerve process, the membrane around the site of the action potential can be divided into three regions. (1) The region in which the action potential is currently generated. (2) The region, just in front of the action potential, that is beginning to be depolarized by the action potential and will soon generate an action potential itself. (3) The region, behind the action potential, that is starting the recovery phase of the action potential, although its sodium channels are still inactivated. This inactivation ensures that the third region will not produce another spike. The region is said to be *refractory* (unable to spike). Inactivation also stops a cell from spiking if it is kept strongly depolarized, a state called *accommodation*.

Depolarization of a neuron increases the probability that a sodium channel will briefly open and that potassium channels will open. Neither of these channel events has a threshold. Then what is meant by threshold for an action potential?

In depolarizations below threshold, the current through potassium channels exceeds the current through sodium channels, so the net effect is a hyperpolarization. At threshold, the sodium current exceeds the potassium current; this causes a depolarization, which activates more channels leading to a further depolarization. This chain reaction (positive feedback) produces the action potential, and it is this point that is threshold.

CABLE PROPERTIES

The enormous computing power of the brain derives from two attributes of neurons, their active channel gating and their passive cable properties.

Because of these properties the voltage change in a neuron is not a simple on–off switch. Cable properties received their name because of the analogy with the electrical properties of transatlantic cables first described by Lord Kelvin. The principle is that current (flow of ions) running along a cable will leak out of the cable in much the same way water will escape from a hose dotted with small holes (Figure 3–8A).

Thus the voltage produced at one point in a neuron will decline as it travels along the nerve fiber (e.g., dendrite).

This means that the response of a neuron depends not only on the size of the stimulus but also on the location of the stimulus along the dendrite. A precise description of the decline of voltage with distance can be complex, but descriptions of simple conditions can provide an intuitive sense of the process.

In a simple case, the voltage declines exponentially with distance (Figure 3–8).

The distance along the dendrite at which the voltage declines to 37% of the original voltage is called the *length constant.*

Thus, the longer the length constant of a dendrite the further a detectable electrical signal can travel. On what properties of the dendrite does the length constant depend? The analogy with the leaky hose may help. The length constant will increase if the membrane resistance (R_m) of the dendrite is high. This is equivalent to patching some of the holes in the hose (more holes, less surface

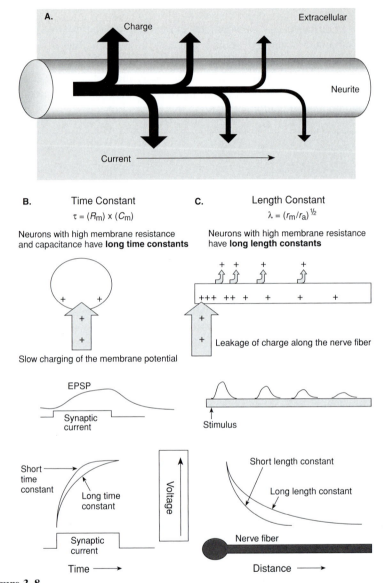

A.

Charge

Extracellular

Neurite

Current

B. Time Constant

$\tau = (R_m) \times (C_m)$

Neurons with high membrane resistance and capacitance have **long time constants**

Slow charging of the membrane potential

EPSP

Synaptic current

Short time constant

Long time constant

Voltage

Synaptic current

Time

C. Length Constant

$\lambda = (r_m/r_a)^{1/2}$

Neurons with high membrane resistance have **long length constants**

Leakage of charge along the nerve fiber

Stimulus

Short length constant

Long length constant

Nerve fiber

Distance

Figure 3–8

(**A**) A graded potential becomes smaller as it propagates along a nerve because some of the charge leaks out of the neuron. (**B, C**) Membrane cable properties and graded potentials. The time constant measures the speed of response of a neuron. In a cell with a long time constant, the graded potential (EPSP) changes slowly. The length constant measures how small the graded potential becomes as it travels along a nerve fiber. In a neuron with a short length constant, the graded potential will become very small after traveling a short distance.

resistance). The length constant will also increase if the diameter of the dendrite is larger. This is equivalent to using a larger hose. Finally, the length constant will increase if the internal resistance (R_i) is low. This is equivalent to a hose with a clean bore, as opposed to a hose that has dirt clinging to the inside (high internal resistance).

Not only is the decline of voltage along the length of a nerve process exponential, but the change of voltage with time is also exponential. This means that a rapid stimulus to a neuron produces a slower voltage response in that neuron.

> The *time constant* is a measure of the speed of response. It is the time it takes for a neuron's response to reach 63% of its final, full response.

The time constant depends on two properties of a neuron, its membrane resistance (which we have already discussed) and its membrane capacitance. Capacitance acts like a reservoir or sponge. If the wall of our leaky hose was made of sponge, the water would have to saturate the sponge before traveling along the dendrite, thus slowing the flow. Capacitance is a property of the lipid membrane that does not change, thus it is a factor not a variable. The membrane resistance is the only variable controlling the time constant. If membrane resistance decreases (more holes in the hose, more open channels in the dendrite), the time constant declines and the nerve responds more quickly.

Related to these cable properties is the speed of conduction of an electrical signal along a nerve process. The speed of propagation is proportional to the square root of the radius. Thus conduction is faster in a larger diameter process.

> Many neuronal processes are constrained by their cable properties, but neurons have evolved mechanisms to overcome these limitations.

The slow time constant of cells has been overcome by *myelination,* which reduces the capacitance and therefore shortens the time constant. Neurons also use voltage-gated channels to boost the response to stimuli, which also speeds up the response. To prevent the decay of the signal with distance, the constraints of the length constant are overcome by the use of action potentials, which act like voltage boosters along the length of a process. The conduction velocity of a signal along a process can be increased by saltatory conduction, through which an action potential jumps rapidly along the axon from one node of Ranvier to the next. Thus, neurons can either take advantage of the cable properties, which are important for signal integration in a neuron, or bypass the limitations of the cable properties by specialized mechanisms.

These cable properties can be expressed mathematically: In a round cell, capacitance makes the voltage response exponential:

$$V(t) = I_m \times R\left(1 - e^{-t/\tau}\right)$$

where I_m is the membrane current, t is time, and τ is the time constant, which is equal to the product of the membrane resistance and capacitance ($\tau = R \times C$). The time constant is the time (in seconds) required for the voltage of the cell to reach 63% ($1/e$; $1/2.7$) of its final value (Figure 3–8). If current is injected at one point, the voltage response of the nerve fiber will be greatest at that point (V_o) and decline exponentially (V_m) with distance (x) from that point.

The *length constant* λ refers to the distance from the point of current injection at which the voltage decreases by 63% of its final value:

$$V_m(x) = V_o e^{-x/\lambda}$$

The length constant is related to the ratio of the membrane and axial resistances:

$$\lambda = \left(r_m/r_a\right)^{\frac{1}{2}}$$

Therefore, the length constant is proportional to the square root of the radius. The length constant is an important factor in spatial summation and saltatory conduction.

SYNAPTIC POTENTIALS

The *synapse* is a specialized structure that permits communication between two cells. There are two types of synapses: chemical and electrical.

An electrical synapse is a physical union between two cells formed by a gap junction. Channel proteins, connexons, on adjoining cells can form a gap junction. When the two connexons link, they can form a pore that acts as a conductor between the cells. Electrical synapses permit very fast communication between cells, but the electrical signal declines as it passes from one cell to another.

This contrasts with the chemical synapse, which is slightly slower but permits much more control of the relationship between the signal in the presynaptic cell and the response in the postsynaptic cell. The events at a chemical synapse are also more complex. The first requirement at a chemical synapse is the depolarization of the presynaptic cell. This depolarization opens voltage-dependent calcium channels. The resulting rise in internal calcium stimulates events leading to fusion of synaptic vesicles with the plasma membrane. This fusion results in extrusion of transmitter into the synaptic space between the pre- and postsynaptic cells. The transmitter rapidly diffuses to the postsynaptic membrane where it binds to specific receptors. This activates the receptors, which results in the opening of receptor channels (ionotropic receptors) or activation of metabolic events (metabotropic receptors). The final event at the synapse is removal of transmitter, either by degradation, diffusion, or reuptake into cells.

Synaptic Plasticity

> The signal across a synapse can be altered by presynaptic and/or postsynaptic mechanisms.

Examples of presynaptic mechanisms are as follows:

Facilitation: An increase in the postsynaptic response resulting from an increase in transmitter release *during* the course of a series of stimuli. Facilitation is due in part to a build-up of calcium in the presynaptic terminal during repetitive stimulation.

Adaptation: A reduction in *response* to maintained stimulation, common in sensory systems. It allows the neuron to be more responsive to changes in stimulation, and increases the dynamic range. Adaptation often results from a calcium-activated potassium conductance.

Autoreceptors: Transmitter released from the presynaptic terminal may affect not only postsynaptic receptors but also presynaptic receptors (Figure 3–9). A transmitter often activates channels on the postsynaptic cell (ionotropic receptors) and at the same time activates metabotropic receptors on the presynaptic membrane that suppress voltage-dependent calcium channels and therefore reduce transmitter release (negative feedback).

Shunting: An inhibitory neuron may synapse onto the presynaptic terminal of a second neuron, preventing the latter cell from releasing transmitter. Two possible mechanisms are involved: (1) closing calcium channels or (2) opening chloride channels. This second mechanism is called shunting. An example is recurrent inhibition in the spinal cord, where Renshaw cells in the spinal cord provide glycinergic negative feedback inhibition to motor neurons.

Potentiation: An increase in synaptic signaling that occurs *following* repetitive stimulation. Potentiation has a slower onset and a longer duration than facilitation. An example is the increase in the response to a single stimulation if it follows a rapid train of stimuli (tetanus). If the potentiation lasts for hours or days it is termed *long-term potentiation* (LTP). The mechanisms for potentiation are

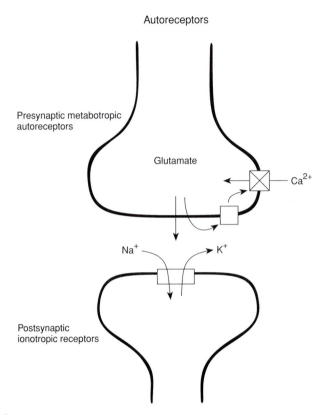

Figure 3–9
At a synapse, the neurotransmitter may affect not only postsynaptic cells but also presynaptic cells that released the transmitter. In this figure, glutamate is released by a presynaptic cell, opening a postsynaptic channel that is permeable to both sodium and potassium. But glutamate also activates a receptor on the presynaptic membrane causing the closure of a calcium channel, thus stopping transmitter release.

varied, including both presynaptic (e.g., an increase in transmitter release) and postsynaptic (e.g., an increase in receptor number).

PRESYNAPTIC MODULATION OF TRANSMITTER RELEASE

Habituation and Sensitization in *Aplysia*

Aplysia, an invertebrate animal, has been very useful in experiments on neuronal plasticity. Stimulation of the siphon sensory neuron activates the gill withdrawal motor neuron. After repetitive stimulation of the siphon sensory neuron there is a reduction in the number of available, presynaptic calcium channels, thereby reducing transmitter release (habituation). Thus, the gill is no longer withdrawn when the siphon is stimulated. After habituation, a novel stimulus (such as a stimulus to the head of the animal) activates an interneuron that synapses on the presynaptic terminal of the siphon sensory neuron, reducing potassium conductance. This prolongs calcium entry and increases transmitter release (sensitization) (Figure 3–10). Under these conditions, once again the gill is withdrawn when the siphon is stimulated.

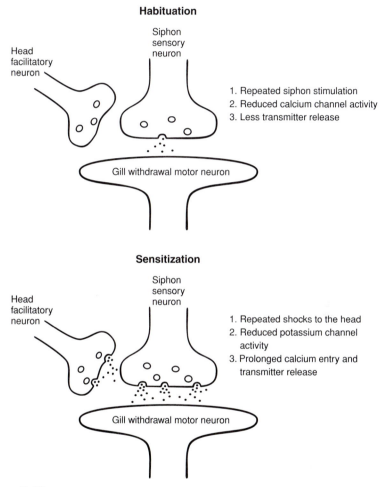

Figure 3–10
In *Aplysia* neurons, stimulation of the siphon causes gill withdrawal. *Habituation:* After repeated siphon stimulation, gill withdrawal subsides. This is a result of a reduction in presynaptic calcium. *Sensitization:* If a novel stimulus is applied to the head of the animal, then a subsequent stimulation of the siphon once again causes gill withdrawal. This is a result of closing of potassium channels on the sensory nerve terminal, allowing a prolonged depolarization and more calcium influx, thus more transmitter release.

POSTSYNAPTIC PLASTICITY

Temporal Summation

If a second excitatory postsynaptic potential (EPSP) arrives at a synapse before the first EPSP ends, the two responses will sum. A longer time constant provides more opportunity for summation.

Spatial Summation

Simultaneous stimulation at two synaptic locations of a neuron will sum. A longer length constant provides more opportunity for summation.

Shunting or Hyperpolarizing Inhibition

Hyperpolarizing inhibition diminishes an EPSP by making the membrane potential more negative. Shunting inhibition may not produce a hyperpolarization, but may still diminish an EPSP. Inhibitory postsynaptic potentials (IPSPs) and EPSPs are not additive, and a small depolarization may still be inhibitory.

Postsynaptic Receptors

Postsynaptic receptors can act simply to open or close channels. But the action of synaptic receptors is often more complex. Two examples are M-current and N-methyl-D-aspartate (NMDA) receptors.

M-Current   Acetylcholine (acting at muscarinic receptors) reduces a voltage-dependent potassium current. This alone does not produce a depolarization, but augments the EPSP produced by other factors.

NMDA Receptors   One receptor stimulated by glutamate is the NMDA receptor. But even when activated by glutamate, this receptor conducts very little depolarizing current unless the neuron is already partially depolarized. This is because magnesium blocks the open NMDA receptor channel when the cell is hyperpolarized. Therefore, NMDA receptor activation is more effective when combined with another EPSP, even if the other EPSP is weak. This has been used as a model of associative learning termed the *Hebbian synapse.*

· C H A P T E R · 4 ·

SYNAPTIC TRANSMISSION
·

Edward Koenig

Types of Synapses

Secretory Pathways

Transduction of an Action Potential into a Chemical Signal

Presynaptic Specializations for Secretion

Molecular Machinery for Membrane Fusion

Retrieval of Vesicular Membrane after Exocytosis

Structure and Properties of the Neuromuscular Synapse

Postsynaptic Events at the Neuromuscular Junction

Diseases of the Neuromuscular Junction

Differences between CNS Synapses and the Neuromuscular Junction

**Motor Neuron as a Model for Excitatory Postsynaptic Potentials
   and Inhibitory Postsynaptic Potentials**

Excitatory and Inhibitory Reflex Pathways to a Motor Neuron

TYPES OF SYNAPSES

> The axon serves as a line of communication that links the nerve cell body to its target cell through a special junction called the synapse.

There are two commonly recognized categories of synapses, electrical and chemical, depending on whether the bioelectrical signal conducted along the axon (i.e., action potential) is transmitted to the target cell by a direct flow of ionic current through the junction (electrical synapse) or whether the bioelectrical signal is first transduced into a chemical signal in the axon terminal, which then acts as a mediator (chemical synapse).

Electrical Synapses

> In an *electrical synapse,* junctional specializations form direct intercellular cytoplasmic channels called *connexons,* through which ionic current can flow from the presynaptic terminal into the postsynaptic cell.

Such synapses are also called *gap junctions* in somatic tissues, and the diffusion of ionic (and nonionic) substances (solutes) across them is nonselective in that the solute need only be less than 1000 Da. Because of direct electrical continuity between pre- and postsynaptic cells, electrical synapses are bidirectional but only sign conserving in nature; that is, the polarity change of the postjunctional cell voltage is always the same as the polarity change of the prejunctional cell voltage (e.g., a presynaptic depolarization does not produce a postsynaptic hyperpolarization). Functionally, this type of synapse often serves to synchronize the activity of a number of cells, and it is found in only a few regions of the central nervous system. Gap junctions in cardiac and smooth muscles serve as intercellular current pathways to depolarize a large population of cells at the same time during conduction of excitation.

Chemical Synapses

The most abundant type of synapse in the nervous system is chemical.

> The *chemical synapse* consists of a close contact between cells that is separated by a *synaptic cleft,* which varies in width depending on whether the synapse is located in the peripheral nervous system (PNS) or in the central nervous system (CNS).

In the PNS, the synaptic cleft is wider because an extracellular matrix, called the *basal lamina,* separates the axon terminal from the postsynaptic cell. In the CNS, there is no extracellular matrix, and the cleft separation is narrower. Any structure or activity before the cleft is referred to as *presynaptic,* and any structure or activity after the cleft is referred to as *postsynaptic.* Because there is no electrical continuity between pre- and postsynaptic cells, a chemical transmitter is required to bridge the cleft space to deliver the signal. The transmitter may mediate either excitation or inhibition, depending on the transmitter and the nature of the receptor/ion channels activated by the transmitter in the membrane of the postsynaptic cell.

> The chemical synapse is structurally polarized so that information can flow in only one direction, from the presynaptic side to the postsynaptic side.

Thus, presynaptic terminals, which are also called *boutons,* contain a population of microvesicles, called *synaptic vesicles,* that stores transmitter. The postsynaptic membrane contains receptors that bind transmitter. Excitatory synapses have a prominent *postsynaptic density.*

SECRETORY PATHWAYS

> There are two types of *secretory pathways* in cells: (1) a *constitutive,* or *unregulated* pathway, which provides membrane constituents for plasma membrane turnover and secretory products for release into the extracellular space, and (2) a *regulated* pathway, which provides secretory products stored in large vesicles that are released in response to an external chemical signal at the cell surface.

In neurons, synaptic vesicles are derived from the constitutive secretory pathway, which is modified in axon terminals because fusion of vesicles with the membrane is ordinarily inhibited by a fusion clamp (Figure 4–1). This results in an accumulation of vesicles (that store transmitter and neuromodulators) in axon terminals that can be released when the fusion clamp is removed by a local increase in intracellular Ca^{2+} concentration.

The vesicles are of different types:

> small neurotransmitter molecules such as *acetylcholine* (ACh), *glutamate* (Glu), *γ-aminobutyric acid* (GABA), and *glycine* (Gly) are stored in small clear synaptic vesicles (diameter: 40–60 nm), and amine neurotransmitters such as *norepinephrine* (NE), *serotonin* (5-HT), and *dopamine* (dopa) are stored in small dense core vesicles (40–60 nm).

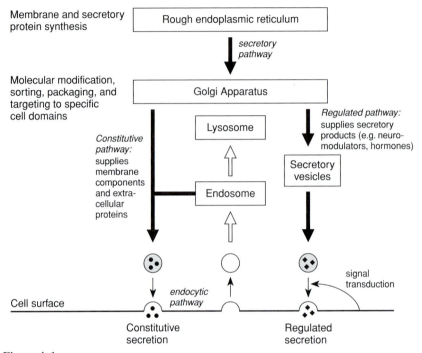

Figure 4–1
Two secretory pathways: constitutive and regulated. Neurotransmitter release involves a modification of the constitutive pathway in which the secretion is fusion clamped until stimulated by calcium influx.

Neuropeptides are stored in medium dense core (80–100 nm) and large dense core vesicles (90–250 nm). Many synaptic terminals may have both clear and dense core vesicles, which means that a transmitter and a neuromodulator can be coreleased. However, dense core vesicles, containing neuromodulators, are located at some distance from the site from which the transmitter is released. As a result a stronger or more sustained stimulation of the presynaptic cell is needed to release the neuromodulator, and the time required for release is longer (e.g., 10 msec for a neuromodulator compared with 0.5 msec for a neurotransmitter).

TRANSDUCTION OF AN ACTION POTENTIAL INTO A CHEMICAL SIGNAL

The *action potential,* which is a transient depolarization of ~0.1 V (100 mV) in amplitude, activates voltage-dependent Ca^{2+} channels in the terminal membrane.

With a $[Ca^{2+}]_o$ (concentration outside) of 1–2 mM and a $[Ca^{2+}]_i$ (concentration inside) of ~10^{-7} M, the very steep electrochemical gradient favors the influx of Ca^{2+} when Ca^{2+} channels are activated. The activation is initiated when the action potential nears its peak. The delay before channels are activated is a major component of the synaptic delay of ~0.5 msec that characterizes chemical transmission in general. Ca^{2+} channels are very close to sites of transmitter release, and this local $[Ca^{2+}]_i$ increases rapidly to high micromolar or even millimolar concentrations, which triggers release of transmitter by removing a Ca^{2+}-sensitive fusion clamp. Dense core vesicles containing neuromodulators are more sensitive to increases in internal calcium, but they are far from this site of calcium entry. Consequently, they do not experience such high concentrations of calcium. The calcium level that they detect is much lower and takes much longer to develop.

It takes 0.1–1 sec for $[Ca^{2+}]_i$ to return to a normal value. Mechanisms for regulating Ca^{2+} in the terminal are summarized in Figure 4–2.

> The short-term mechanism for lowering $[Ca^{2+}]_i$ occurs by diffusion and uptake into a *smooth endoplasmic reticulum* (SER) in the presynaptic terminal.

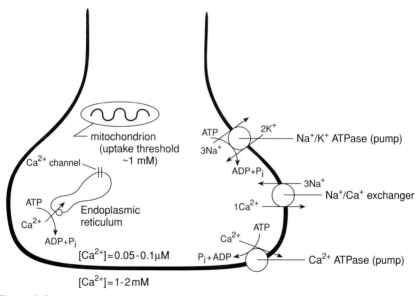

Figure 4–2
Control of calcium concentration in the presynaptic terminal. Calcium is actively pumped into the endoplasmic reticulum and out of the cell. It is also removed from the cell by an Na^+/Ca^{2+} exchanger that gets its energy from the Na^+ gradient produced by the Na^+/K^+ pump. Mitochondria may also take up calcium if levels in the cell become high.

Uptake into SER is promoted by a high-affinity, low-capacity adenosine tri-phosphate (ATP)-dependent Ca^{2+} pump in the SER membrane. Although mito-chondria in the terminal can also take up Ca^{2+}, it is a low-affinity (~1 mM), high-capacity system that comes into play when $[Ca^{2+}]_i$ becomes very high.

> Long-term regulation of $[Ca^{2+}]_i$ involves extrusion of Ca^{2+} by a high-affinity, low-capacity ATP-dependent plasma membrane (PM) Ca^{2+} pump and an Na^+/Ca^{2+} exchanger on the PM.

The exchanger is a low-affinity, high-capacity system in which three Na^+ ions enter in exchange for one Ca^{2+} extruded. Na^+ ions are then extruded in exchange for K^+ by the PM Na^+/K^+ pump in a ratio of 3:2, respectively.

PRESYNAPTIC SPECIALIZATIONS FOR SECRETION

> Transmitter is released from restricted sites in the terminal PM facing the synaptic cleft, called *active zones,* and voltage-gated Ca^{2+} channels are located in the immediate vicinity.

Synaptic vesicles, which store the transmitter, are predocked at the active zones. The predocked and nearby undocked vesicles belong to a so-called read-ily releasable pool of synaptic vesicles that represents an immediately available source of transmitter. A larger reserve pool of vesicles is not free to move because it is tethered to a cytoskeletal network, made up primarily of *synapsin,* which links the vesicle to *filamentous (F) actin* of the cell's cytoskeleton. Tethering and release of vesicles from the network are regulated by synapsin, an 80-kDa protein that has a globular head and a collagen-like tail. In the dephosphorylated state, it binds tightly to vesicles and to actin filaments. Phosphorylation of synapsin by Ca^{2+}/calmodulin-dependent kinase II (CaMKII) causes dissociation of vesicles from the tether. Thus, vesicles can be mobilized from the reserve pool with sus-tained neural activity. That is,

> as $[Ca^{2+}]_i$ increases and CaMKII is activated, synapsin becomes phosphory-lated, the cytoskeletal tether disassembles, and vesicles can be mobilized to active zones.

Details of the machinery and mechanisms governing the actual release of transmitter from the terminal are only partially understood. Synaptic vesicles are recycled, so that after emptying their contents, they are recharged or reprimed with transmitter.

There appear to be two forms of transmitter release from vesicles: *exocytosis* and formation of a *fusion pore.*

In the first case, release of transmitter occurs when a docked vesicle fuses completely with the PM to release its contents by exocytosis. In the second case, the vesicle forms a temporary, small connection with the PM, a fusion pore. This pore forms transiently in the PM and serves as a channel for transmitter release into the synaptic cleft. In the former case, the membrane would have to be retrieved to reform a vesicle, and in the latter case, the vesicle would simply dissociate from the PM. The fusion clamp, which inhibits unregulated transmitter release, is removed by a local increase in $[Ca^{2+}]_i$ at the active zone. These events are summarized in Figure 4–3.

Overview of Transmitter Release Events

1. Vesicles must be predocked at active zone
2. Ca^{2+} channels must be within 10 nm of fusion site
3. Unregulated fusion is inhibited until Ca^{2+} enters

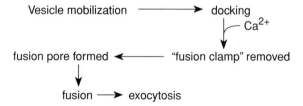

Figure 4–3
Cycle of transmitter release. Synaptic vesicles are moved to docking sites but are not released due to a fusion clamp. Calcium influx removes the clamp, leading to transmitter release.

MOLECULAR MACHINERY FOR MEMBRANE FUSION

Cells have many intracellular membrane-enclosed compartments [e.g., rough endoplasmic reticulum (RER), SER, Golgi complex, lysosomes, and endosomes] in which specific metabolic functions are performed.

Secretory cargo and/or membrane components are transferred from one compartment to another via vesicles. Docking of a vesicle to its target membrane is a prerequisite to fusion, which depends on a specific membrane–membrane interaction.

The basic mechanisms that mediate specific membrane interactions are explained by the *SNARE hypothesis* (Figure 4–4), which seeks to elucidate the molecular events responsible for vesicle docking, priming, fusion, and recovery.

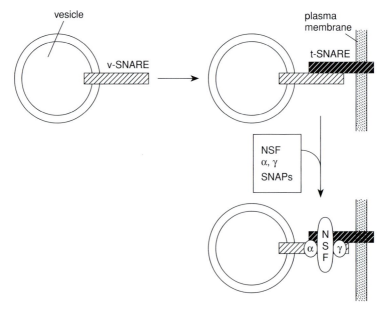

Figure 4–4
SNARE hypothesis. Proteins associated with the vesicle (v-SNAREs) and with the plasma membrane (t-SNAREs) interact to promote docking, fusion, neurotransmitter release, and vesicle recycling. NSF, N-ethylmaleimide-sensitive factor.

A vesicle-associated membrane protein (*VAMP*) serves as a *v-SNARE*, which can recognize and bind to the PM by forming a docking complex with the cognate target membrane *t-SNARE*. The basic docking complex is made up of *synaptobrevin,* the v-SNARE of the vesicle membrane, and *syntaxin,* the cognate *t-SNARE* in the synaptic PM. There are many other important proteins in both the PM, such as *SNAP-25* (a synaptosomal-associated protein of 25 kDa), and the vesicle membrane, such as synaptotagmin and Rab3. Neurotoxins, such as tetanus and botulinum toxins, block transmitter release by proteolytic cleavage of one or more docking complex proteins (i.e., synaptobrevin, syntaxin, and SNAP-25).

Initially, as mentioned previously, the vesicle is locked in the reserve pool because of the action of synapsin. After release from the reserve pool, the vesicle can approach and dock at the presynaptic terminal. Before docking can occur a blocking protein, Sec1, has to be removed from the t-SNARE. This is accomplished by Rab3, a vesicle-associated low-molecular-weight guanine nucleotide–binding protein that is involved in vesicle docking.

> *Rab3* is believed to regulate the speed of assembly of SNARE complexes by displacing *Sec1* from the t-SNARE, permitting formation of a docking complex between the t-SNARE and the v-SNARE.

Thus, guanosine triphosphate (GTP)-bound Rab3 modulates the rate of membrane docking by promoting the formation of docking complexes.

When attached to a vesicle, Rab3 is also complexed with rabphilin, a Rab3 effector protein. After the vesicle fusion event, Rab3-bound GTP is hydrolyzed to guanosine diphosphate (GDP) and inorganic phosphate (P_i), catalyzed by a GTPase-activating protein (GAP). This causes rabphilin to dissociate, and GDP–Rab3 is removed from the vesicle membrane by a protein called GDP dissociation inhibitor (GDI). In the dissociated state, GDP is exchanged for GTP, which is catalyzed by a GDP–GTP exchange protein. GTP–Rab3 can then reassociate with free vesicles and bind rabphilin for another docking cycle.

> Additional components of the fusion machinery include *N*-ethylmaleimide-sensitive factor (*NSF*), a homotrimer with ATPase activity, and α- and γ-*SNAP* proteins, which are soluble proteins.

The α- and γ-SNAP proteins are required for NSF binding to the SNARE complex. Although the role of SNAP/NSF proteins is not entirely clear, they are required for multiple rounds of fusion under physiological conditions. NSF serves to alter the SNARE complex and may be the event that produces vesicle priming, a metastable, membrane-attached state of the vesicle. A recent suggestion is that SNAP/NSF proteins promote disassembly of the SNARE complex and release of vesicle after fusion, which would require ATP hydrolysis by NSF. Once the vesicle is primed at the active zone, calcium influx initiates fusion. The voltage-dependent calcium channel is tethered close to the release site by syntaxin. This ensures that there will be a high local level of internal calcium. Although the mechanism by which Ca^{2+} triggers fusion is unknown, *synaptotagmin,* another vesicle protein, may be the Ca^{2+} sensor because it has two regulatory low-affinity Ca^{2+} binding domains, and it also binds syntaxin, the t-SNARE, in a Ca^{2+}-dependent manner. The mechanism of fusion, however, is poorly understood.

RETRIEVAL OF VESICULAR MEMBRANE AFTER EXOCYTOSIS

Neuronal synaptic transmission is an extremely rapid event compared with regulated secretion in nonneural cells, because of predocking and priming of vesicles and the very close proximity of voltage-gated Ca^{2+} channels to fusion sites. A typical presynaptic terminal in the CNS may contain only 200 synaptic vesicles.

> Ongoing neuronal activity would rapidly deplete the vesicular content if vesicles were not rapidly and efficiently recycled.

One model for replenishing synaptic vesicles suggests that vesicles form a transient fusion pore through which transmitter is released; vesicles would reseal while dissociating from the active zone and could then be recharged with transmitter for another round of release. Although this would be a rapid and energy-efficient mechanism, evidence for it is limited.

> The traditional view for recycling synaptic vesicles assumes that the vesicle membrane fuses completely with the PM, a process called *exocytosis,* and is then retrieved from the PM by a process called *endocytosis,* which is driven by an energy-dependent membrane retrieval machinery.

The retrieval machinery is known to be expressed in nerve cells at levels that are 10–15 times greater than in nonneural cells.

> Several components are involved in retrieval of vesicular membrane and recycling pathway: (1) *clathrin,* a coat assembly protein that becomes attached to the membrane patch to be endocytosed, (2) the clathrin adaptor proteins *AP2* and *AP3,* (3) *dynamin,* a large guanine nucleotide–binding protein that promotes endocytosis of the coated membrane, and (4) *hsc70,* a clathrin uncoating ATPase.

Depolarization initiates synaptic vesicle recycling, and the first step in the process is the appearance of an internalization signal on the cytoplasmic surface of the exocytosed membrane patch. This signal is believed to be the cytoplasmic domain of synaptotagmin. AP2 complexes bind to synaptotagmin and recruit AP3 complexes, which promote clathrin coat assembly. An elevation in $[Ca^{2+}]_i$ leads to activation of *calcineurin,* a phosphatase that dephosphorylates dynamin. The dephosphorylated dynamin initiates endocytosis by the invagination and pinching off of the coated membrane. Hsc70 promotes clathrin uncoating, and the vesicle takes up transmitter and can enter the readily releasable or reserve vesicle pools. Salient features of this are summarized in Figure 4–5.

Endocytotic phase adapted to presynaptic terminals

1. Typical CNS terminal has only 200 vesicles
2. Latency for membrane retrieval is very brief
3. Retrieval machinery is expressed 10- to 15-fold higher than in nonneural cells

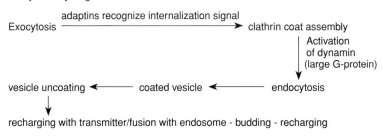

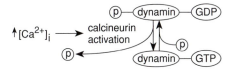

Figure 4–5
Endocytosis. Vesicles are re-formed after removal from the membrane by clathrin coat assembly and dynamin activation.

STRUCTURE AND PROPERTIES
OF THE NEUROMUSCULAR SYNAPSE

One of the best studied synapses is the neuromuscular junction. Myofibers in skeletal muscles, which are controlled by motor neurons, are large, elongated, multinucleated cells that are many tens of microns in diameter.

> The functional *motor unit* consists of one motor neuron and all the myofibers that it innervates.

Motor units can range in size from a few myofibers in muscles that require fine control (e.g., ocular, laryngeal, ear ossicle movements) to several hundred myofibers in powerful force-generating muscles.

> The transmitter at the neuromuscular junction is *acetylcholine* (ACh), which is excitatory when it binds to ionotropic acetylcholine receptors in the postsynaptic membrane.

Such acetylcholine receptors are classified as *nicotinic* receptors, because nicotine is an agonist (see below). Transmission is highly reliable unless there is an underlying pathology; that is, one nerve action potential always evokes a muscle action potential. The large myofiber, compared with the motor axon, requires a large influx of ionic current (i.e., a large increase in conductance) to bring about membrane depolarization. This is achieved by the large surface area of synaptic contact, because

> the surface area governs the number of presynaptic transmitter release sites, called *active zones,* and the number of postsynaptic ionotropic receptors available to bring about a change in conductance.

This illustrates one distinction between the synapses between neurons and the synapses between motor neurons and skeletal muscle fibers. A single muscle fiber has only one synaptic site, at which a presynaptic neuron releases a large number of vesicles. In connections between two neurons, there are usually multiple synaptic sites, but only one vesicle, or a few vesicles, is released per site.

Motor axon terminals lie in groove-like invaginations at the surface of the myofiber, in which the postsynaptic PM contains infoldings. Areas of close contact between pre- and postsynaptic membranes form a *primary cleft,* and postsynaptic membrane infoldings form a *secondary cleft.* A basal lamina occupies the space in primary and secondary clefts. Presynaptic terminals contain a large population of ~40-nm synaptic vesicles, each of which stores 5000 to 10,000 acetylcholine molecules (quantal size).

> The content of one vesicle, which is released into the synaptic cleft, comprises one *quantum* of transmitter, and a quantum can be released from each of the many active zones in a terminal.

In response to a single nerve action potential, a total of 200–300 quanta are released into the synaptic cleft. Repetitive stimulation of an afferent nerve, called *tetanus,* produces an increase in the number of quanta released (i.e., quantal content). This results in an enhancement in the postsynaptic potential, which is called *facilitation.* It is the result of insufficient time to remove residual Ca^{2+} left over from previous action potentials.

> Synaptic transmission at the *neuromuscular junction* (NMJ) can be suppressed experimentally so that only one quantam, or at most a few quanta, is released when the motor neuron is stimulated.

The postsynaptic response under these conditions is not an end-plate potential (EPP), but a miniature EPP or mEPP. The mEPP may be 0.5 mV, 1 mV, 1.5 mV, etc., that is, it is a multiple of a basic unit of 0.5 mV. Thus, a single vesicle releases a quantum of transmitter, and each quantum produces a depolarization of about 0.5 mV.

The active zones are strategically located over the crests of the postsynaptic folds, where acetylcholine receptors (AChRs) are localized in a high density of $10,000/\mu m^2$. An electron-dense undercoating at the top of the folds is due to a cytoskeletal matrix that anchors AChR channels so that they are immobilized.

> Anchored in the basal lamina of the synaptic clefts is *acetylcholinesterase* (AChE), the enzyme that terminates transmitter action by hydrolyzing acetylcholine into acetate and choline.

Choline is then taken up into the presynaptic terminal for resynthesis of acetylcholine.

Termination of transmitter action by an enzyme is unique, because the action of most other transmitters in the CNS is terminated by diffusion and rapid uptake by the presynaptic terminal and glial cell processes that surround the synapse.

When ACh is first released from the presynaptic terminal, a portion of it is hydrolyzed by AChE before the ACh ever reaches the receptor. However, there is a very high level of ACh is the cleft, which temporarily overwhelms the degradative effect of AChE. This is sufficient for only one binding event with AChRs of ~1 msec in duration, after which ACh dissociates from the receptor and is hydrolyzed by AChE.

When AChE is inhibited by reversible or irreversible anticholinesterase agents, such as *physiostigmine* (*eserine*) or *organophosphorus* compounds, respectively, multiple ACh-binding events occur, resulting in a prolongation of transmitter action.

Under these conditions diffusion alone terminates transmitter action. It is interesting to note that these AChE inhibitors have been used as nerve gases in wartime. They prevent the termination of muscle excitation, causing asphyxiation and paralysis. However, AChE inhibitors are used to treat patients suffering from myasthenia gravis. In this disease, there is a reduction of ACh receptors, so extending the lifetime of ACh is beneficial.

POSTSYNAPTIC EVENTS AT THE NEUROMUSCULAR JUNCTION

The reaction scheme and sequence of postsynaptic events are as follows:

$$2ACh + AChR \leftrightarrow AChR + ACh \leftrightarrow (ACh)_2R^* \text{ (activated channel)} \rightarrow$$
$$\text{increased end-plate membrane conductance } (\Uparrow g_{EP}) \rightarrow$$
$$\text{net inward end-plate current} \rightarrow \text{end-plate potential (EPP)}$$

Two ACh are required for efficient activation of the receptor. This is a common feature of ionotropic receptors, and it enhances their sensitivity to small changes in transmitter concentration (increases the slope of the dose–response curve). The EPP produces a local circuit current (graded potential) that depolarizes the muscle membrane around the end plate. This depolarization activates voltage-gated Na^+ channels. When threshold is reached, a muscle action potential is generated.

> The ionic basis of the EPP is a nonspecific increase in membrane conductance to both sodium and potassium through AChR channels [i.e., $\uparrow(g_{Na+} + g_{K+})$], in which both cation currents flow through the same channels.

The initial inward current is carried by Na^+ ($-I_{Na+}$), which exceeds the outward K^+ current ($+I_{K+}$) because of differences in the corresponding driving forces on the two cations (i.e., initially the resting membrane potential is closer to E_{K+} than it is to E_{Na+}). This depolarizes the end-plate region. As the membrane depolarizes, the driving force on Na^+ decreases and the driving force on K^+ increases until the two opposing currents become equal at a membrane potential of about -15 mV, which is called the reversal potential (V_r or V_{EPP}). Normally, this depolarization is sufficient to activate an action potential in the muscle fiber. In the meantime, ACh dissociates from AChRs, and channels close. If the muscle action potential is blocked, the EPP decays back to the resting membrane potential due to a different set of potassium channels, often referred to as membrane leakage channels (i.e., nongated K^+ channels) (Figure 4–6).

> *Agonists,* which activate AChR channels, include ACh, *succinylcholine,* and *nicotine. Antagonists,* which bind AChRs but do not activate channels, include *curare*-like drugs such as *d-tubocurarine,* which compete with ACh for binding to AChRs.

Because of competitive binding, curare concentration can be graded to reduce the EPP amplitude below threshold. α-*Bungarotoxin* (BTX), a peptide toxin in snake venom, binds AChRs irreversibly.

> Continued exposure of AChRs to an agonist produces *desensitization,* a condition in which the ligand binds with high affinity, but the channels are in a nonconducting state.

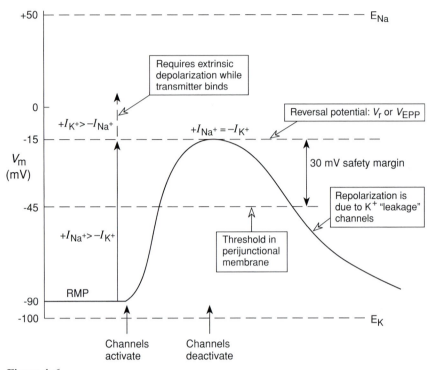

Figure 4–6
Ionic basis of the end-plate potential (EPP). Acetylcholine release from the presynaptic terminal activates channels that are permeable to sodium and potassium. This produces a depolarization to about −15 mV. Then transmitter dissociates because of lower affinity and is hydrolyzed, the channels deactivate, and the muscle cell repolarizes due to the resting (leakage) potassium channels. RMP, resting membrane potential.

For example, because succinylcholine is hydrolyzed very slowly, it will initially produce depolarization of the end plate. But with time, AChRs will become desensitized, and the muscle will repolarize but will be incapable of producing an EPP. However, direct electrical stimulation of the muscle will still generate an action potential, indicating that the spike-generating mechanism is intact, but that the synapse was inactivated. The desensitizing blockade is reversible, and for this reason it has been used as a muscle relaxant during surgery. However, artificial respiration is required.

DISEASES OF THE NEUROMUSCULAR JUNCTION

Myasthenia gravis, an autoimmune disease that is caused by antibodies to the AChR, is a muscle weakness, and sustained effort increases the weakness.

Neuromuscular transmission is impaired and leads to failure to generate action potentials in a variable number of myofibers of each motor unit. Ordinarily, the EPP produces a depolarization that exceeds the threshold for the action potential in myofibers by 35–40 mV, which serves as a margin of safety to ensure that each nerve action potential will produce a muscle action potential. The safety margin is reduced or lost in myasthenia gravis. In an electromyogram this manifests as variations in the amplitudes of compound muscle action potentials caused by the failure of myofibers in various motor units to reach threshold in response to stimulation of the motor nerve.

The pathology includes a widening of the primary synaptic cleft and loss of secondary cleft infoldings and a loss of AChRs. As a consequence the diffusion path of acetylcholine is longer, and fewer AChRs are available to produce the necessary membrane conductance needed to generate a normal EPP. As mentioned, AChE inhibitors can be used to prolong the lifetime of ACh in the cleft, thereby increasing the EPP.

Another disease of the neuromuscular junction is called the *Lambert–Eaton myasthenic syndrome,* which is also a muscle weakness. Unlike myasthenia gravis, the pathology is presynaptic, and a sustained muscle effort improves muscle activity. It is an autoimmune disease that may be associated with oat cell carcinoma of the lung, affecting a specific type of Ca^{2+} channel in the terminal. Thus, a nerve action potential produces a reduced Ca^{2+} conductance ($g_{Ca^{2+}}$), which results in a reduction in the number of quanta released. Repetitive stimulation of the nerve increases quantal content because of a build-up of residual $[Ca^{2+}]$ inside the presynaptic terminal.

DIFFERENCES BETWEEN CNS SYNAPSES AND THE NEUROMUSCULAR JUNCTION

Every myofiber is innervated by a single motor axon that produces excitation and muscle contraction in a highly reliable manner. In contrast, neurons in the CNS may have tens of thousands of presynaptic boutons forming synapses on their surfaces.

> Major types of synapses are *axosomatic, axodendritic* (which include synapses on dendritic shafts and on dendritic spines), and *axoaxonic.*

Spine synapses are excitatory, whereas most axoaxonic synapses are inhibitory; all other synapses may be either excitatory or inhibitory. CNS synapses are stabilized by cell–cell adhesion molecules that cross-link pre- and postsynaptic membranes to form a cleft space of ~15 nm, compared with ~50 nm at the neuromuscular junction.

Synapses are classified into two broad categories: *gray type 1* and *gray type 2.*

Gray 1 synapses have 50-nm round vesicles in presynaptic terminals and are asymmetric with a prominent postsynaptic density. They are excitatory in function, and postsynaptic densities are composed of a cytoskeletal meshwork that anchors excitatory ionotropic receptor channels in the postsynaptic membrane. The meshwork is coated with approximately 30 globular proteins that make up a molecular machinery that plays a role in long-term synaptic modification, such as postsynaptic potentiation.

Postsynaptic potentiation (PTP) is an augmented synaptic potential that is produced at most excitatory synapses in response to a high-frequency tetanus of afferents, in which the potentiated *excitatory postsynaptic potential* remains above normal even after a period of rest.

Gray 2 synapses are symmetric, with scanty postsynaptic density, and are inhibitory in function. Presynaptic vesicles are 40 nm and appear flattened after glutaraldehyde fixation.

MOTOR NEURON AS A MODEL FOR EXCITATORY POSTSYNAPTIC POTENTIALS AND INHIBITORY POSTSYNAPTIC POTENTIALS

Basic definitions related to spinal cord organization include the following:

1. A *motor nucleus* is a population of motor neurons in spinal cord gray matter that innervates a particular muscle.
2. A *motor neuron pool* is a population of motor neuron nuclei in the spinal cord that controls the same function, such as flexion or extension of a joint.
3. *Interneurons,* also called *local circuit neurons* because they are cellular elements in local neural circuits, have short axons, substantially outnumber motor neurons, and are either excitatory or inhibitory. Most afferent inputs to motor neurons are via interneurons, with one exception (see below).

EXCITATORY AND INHIBITORY REFLEX PATHWAYS TO A MOTOR NEURON

The excitatory pathway to a motor neuron may be *monosynaptic* (one synapse) or *polysynaptic* (two or more synapses).

An inhibitory pathway requires at least two synapses, in which an inhibitory neuron is the last in the pathway to synapse with the motor neuron. The single monosynaptic input to motor neurons is from large-diameter *Ia* afferents originating from *stretch receptors* in the same muscle innervated by the motor neuron.

Stimulation of Ia afferents produces a local, decrementing synaptic potential similar to the EPP, called an *excitatory postsynaptic potential (EPSP).*

The EPSP amplitude depends on *spatial summation* and *temporal summation* of active afferents. Spatial summation is produced by simultaneous stimulation of many afferents distributed on the neuron's surface. Temporal summation is produced when a given number of afferents is stimulated repetitively, such that each succeeding action potential in the afferents produces another EPSP before previous EPSPs decay completely. The region of lowest threshold is the axon hillock–initial axon segment, which is called the *action potential trigger zone,* in which there is a high density of voltage-gated Na^+ channels in the membrane.

The ionic basis of the EPSP is similar to the EPP; that is, there is a nonspecific increase in membrane conductance to monovalent cations [i.e., $\uparrow$ (g_{Na^+} + g_{K^+})]; however, unlike the neuromuscular junction, V_r or V_{EPSP} is 0 mV. The net inward synaptic current (I_{EPSP}) at active excitatory synapses generates an EPSP, resulting in a local circuit current that depolarizes the surrounding membrane. If depolarization reaches threshold at the action potential trigger zone, a nerve action potential is generated. Because synaptic potentials are decrementing graded potentials, synapses closest to the action potential trigger zone are more effective than those farther away.

The most common excitatory transmitter in the central nervous system is *glutamate.* Glutamate is the probable transmitter for most CNS excitatory synapses including most primary sensory nerve endings, but there are multiple receptors.

Glutamate binds to three types of receptors: *Q-type* (the specific agonist is *quisqualate*), *K-type* (the specific agonist is *kainate*), and *NMDA* (the specific agonist is *N-methyl-D-aspartate*).

Q- and K-type receptors mediate transmission at most excitatory synapses. NMDA receptors (NMDARs) are noteworthy because these synapses are modifiable and are presumably involved in memory mechanisms. They have the following unique properties: (1) Mg^{2+} lodges in the channels and blocks the increase in conductance through the channel when NMDARs are activated while the cell is at its resting membrane potential (RMP). Conductance through the NMDAR channel occurs when simultaneous activation of synapses with Q and/or K receptor channels depolarizes the membrane, which ejects Mg^{2+} from the channel; and (2) Ca^{2+}, Na^+, and K^+ currents flow through activated NMDAR channels. Ca^{2+} also acts as an intracellular second messenger to trigger biochemical pathways that affect long-term modification of synapses (e.g., long-term potentiation).

Termination of transmitter action is by Na^+-dependent uptake of transmitter by presynaptic terminals and by neighboring glial cell processes that surround synapses.

Glutamate is toxic in high concentrations. Glutamate toxicity kills neurons and may cause cell damage by excessive excitation, as during persistent grand mal seizures or after ischemia from a stroke. Cell death is a result of multiple factors, including abnormally high $[Ca^{2+}]_i$ due to activation of NMDAR channels, which overwhelm mechanisms for intracellular Ca^{2+} buffering. Excessive Ca^{2+} activates proteases and promotes production of chemically reactive free radicals.

Stimulation of an inhibitory pathway generates a *hyperpolarizing inhibitory postsynaptic potential (IPSP)*.

The ionic basis for IPSPs in vertebrates is an increase in membrane conductance to Cl^-. E_{Cl^-} is -80 mV, which is the reversal potential for the IPSP (i.e., E_{IPSP}). If RMP is -70 mV, activation of inhibitory synapses produces an inward Cl^- flux ($+I_{Cl^-}$). At some synapses in invertebrates, the ionic basis of the IPSP is an outward K^+ current ($+I_{K^+}$). In either case, an increased g_{Cl^-} or g_{K^+} hyperpolarizes the membrane.

Although there are inhibitory synapses on dendrites, they tend to concentrate on the cell body, where, being nearer to the action potential trigger zone, they are effective in decreasing excitability. In one mechanism of inhibition the membrane resistance (R_m) on the cell body is decreased, so that local circuit current from excitatory synapses located out on dendrites is shunted (leaks out across the PM) if inhibitory synapses are simultaneously active on the cell body (i.e., effectively decreases λ). This makes current from excitatory synapses less effective in depolarizing the action potential trigger zone. In a second mechanism the IPSP drives the membrane potential toward E_{Cl^-}, and away from E_{Na^+}.

> Common inhibitory transmitters are *glycine* and *γ-aminobutyric acid (GABA)*.

Glycine mediates postsynaptic inhibition in spinal cord and brainstem motor centers, and GABA mediates presynaptic inhibition in spinal cord and brainstem and postsynaptic inhibition elsewhere in the brain. Termination of transmitter action is by uptake into presynaptic terminals and glial processes surrounding the synapse. Antagonists that block transmission, such as *strychnine* for glycine and *picrotoxin* or *biccuculine* for GABA, are potent convulsants. This indicates that neurons are normally under tonic inhibition.

> EPSPs and IPSPs generate opposing local circuit currents.

Thus, the probability of generating nerve action potentials when excitatory and inhibitory synapses are simultaneously active depends on whether there is a sufficient net depolarizing current at the action potential trigger zone to reach threshold. Each synaptic input produces a very small EPSP or IPSP. Thus, in the case of a motor neuron, there are 20,000–50,000 synapses that govern motor neuron output (i.e., frequency of nerve action potentials). Most synapses (~80%) are located on dendrites, with the remaining located on the cell body. If a unitary EPSP on the cell body is ~0.1 mV, RMP is −70 mV, and threshold is −50 mV, a depolarization of 20 mV is required to reach threshold. In this case, a minimum of 200 simultaneously active excitatory synapses would be required to reach threshold.

NEUROTRANSMITTERS

·

Jerome Roth

Methods of Communication

Criteria for a Substance Being a Neurotransmitter

Blood–Brain Barrier: Protector of Brain

Structure and Function of the Synapse

Neurotransmitters and Neuromodulators

Biochemistry of Biogenic Amines

Synthesis and Degradation of Acetylcholine

Synthesis and Degradation of γ-Aminobutyric Acid (GABA)

Synthesis and Degradation of Glutamate

Synthesis and Degradation of Glycine

Neuropeptides

· · · · · · · · · · · ·

METHODS OF COMMUNICATION

The propagation of nerve impulses is a fundamental process that must occur rapidly and be highly discriminative. Communication between neurons is a dynamic event that is regulated by a complex series of positive and negative feedback processes.

> There are basically two mechanisms by which nerve impulses are propagated between neurons. Neuronal cells can communicate electrically through *gap junctions* or chemically by the actions of *neurotransmitters* and *neuromodulators.*

The release of neurotransmitters from nerve terminals and their diffusion across the synaptic cleft to their site of action on the postsynaptic membrane must be a rapid event allowing for highly sensitive and specific regulation of signal transmission between neurons. The effect of the neurotransmitter on binding to its postsynaptic cell membrane receptor can either be excitatory or inhibitory, depending on its polarization of the membrane potential.

> *Excitatory neurotransmitters* decrease polarity across the membrane (depolarize) and, thus, augment the potential for signal propagation in the postsynaptic neurons. *Inhibitory neurotransmitters,* in contrast, increase polarity (hyperpolarize) and prevent the propagation of the action potential.

The specificity of a particular neurotransmitter (whether it acts in an excitatory or inhibitory fashion) is normally an inherent property of the transmitter itself. But it also depends on the functional characteristics of the receptor and the signal transduction pathway to which it is coupled. Thus, neurotransmitters have the potential to initiate different biological responses depending on the specificity of the neuronal system.

This chapter presents a review of the most relevant information regarding the properties and function of the different neurotransmitter systems present in the central nervous system (CNS). It also presents a review of the blood–brain barrier, which is required to protect the brain against exposure to potentially toxic endogenous and exogenous agents.

CRITERIA FOR A SUBSTANCE BEING A NEUROTRANSMITTER

Although large numbers of endogenous chemicals are found in the CNS, only a few of them actually serve in the process of neuronal transmission. Several criteria must be met to classify a substance as a true neurotransmitter as opposed to a neuromodulator or a substance possessing other biological activity. However, before discussing the specific criteria used to establish a chemical as a neurotransmitter, it is first necessary to describe and define the term *neuromodulator*. Unlike a neurotransmitter,

a *neuromodulator* is a substance that by itself has no intrinsic activity in regard to altering membrane potential. Instead, it is a substance that modulates the functions or efficacy of a neurotransmitter.

Thus, in the absence of the actual neurotransmitter, a neuromodulator alone will not induce a response on the postsynaptic membrane. There are a variety of mechanisms by which a substance can act as a neuromodulator. A neuromodulator may alter the binding affinity of a neurotransmitter to its receptor or modulate the signal induced on binding of the neurotransmitter to its receptor. Neuromodulators can also influence synthesis, release, degradation, and storage of neurotransmitters.

Four criteria are used to identify substances as *neurotransmitters* and to distinguish them from neuromodulators:

presence, release, identity of action, and *removal.*

Presence

For a substance to be considered a neurotransmitter, it must be shown to be present in the presynaptic nerve terminal.

In addition, it is likely that this substance will be unevenly distributed in different areas of the brain. Along with this, we expect that synthesizing enzymes for this neurotransmitter will also be present in the neuron and that membrane receptors will be present at the synapse. Although these are essential criteria, they are not sufficient to define a substance as a neurotransmitter because a neuro-modulator can satisfy this definition as well.

Release

> For a substance to be considered a neurotransmitter it must be released in physiologically relevant quantities on nerve stimulation.

Here again, although this is an important and necessary criterion, it is not sufficiently rigorous to define a substance as a neurotransmitter because neuro-modulators can similarly be released in physiologically relevant quantities from presynaptic nerve endings on nerve stimulation. In fact, neuromodulators are often present in the storage vesicle along with the neurotransmitter and are released into the synaptic cleft on nerve stimulation.

Identity of Action

On release of a neurotransmitter and subsequent binding to its receptor, a specific response in the postsynaptic cell occurs.

> For a substance to be considered a neurotransmitter, direct application of this substance to the synapse must produce a response in the postsynaptic neuron similar to that generated on nerve stimulation.

In a related fashion, drugs that alter neurotransmitter function when added to the synapse should alter the action of the applied substance in a manner similar to that observed on nerve stimulation. This criterion is very important as it dis-tinguishes a neurotransmitter from a neuromodulator. In the case of the neuro-modulator, its direct application to the synapse will not induce a response at the postsynaptic membrane.

Removal

> For a substance to be considered a neurotransmitter a mechanism must be present within the synapse that is responsible for the rapid inactivation or removal of active substances.

This process of functional inactivation has to occur extracellularly within the synaptic cleft. It can result either from the release of enzymes into the synaptic cleft that rapidly degrade and inactivate the substance or via a selective reuptake process that rapidly and efficiently removes the substance from the cleft. Although the latter process does not result in the actual inactivation of the substance, it does bring about the rapid and selective removal of the agent from functionally active postsynaptic receptor sites. Once inside the presynaptic nerve terminal, other degradative processes can occur that ultimately inactivate the neurotransmitter.

BLOOD–BRAIN BARRIER: PROTECTOR OF BRAIN

Many of the neurotransmitters and neuromodulators found in the CNS are present in the peripheral circulatory system. Obviously, the CNS needs to be protected from these circulating bioactive agents so that the normal and discriminative processing of information by the different neurotransmitter systems can occur. In this regard, studies as early as 1901 demonstrated that dyes such as trypan blue, when injected intravenously, did not enter the brain. From these seminal studies, the physical existence of the blood–brain barrier was established.

> The *blood–brain barrier* is composed of a lipid-permeable barrier that allows the facile diffusion of lipid-soluble molecules into the brain but selectively impedes the penetration of water-soluble agents into the CNS.

Composition of the Blood–Brain Barrier

Structurally the blood–brain barrier consists of endothelial cells that comprise the blood vessel wall. Surrounding the endothelium is a basement membrane composed of the extracellular matrix protein, collagen. Compared with endothelium in other organs, the brain endothelium has several unique features that account for its performance as a selective barrier preventing water-soluble agents from entering the brain. The most important of these is that

> brain endothelium forms tight junctions preventing passage of molecules between individual cells.

Thus, for substances to penetrate the CNS, they actually have to pass through endothelial cells. This is important, as the metabolic capacity of the brain endothelial cell is considerably greater than the metabolic capacity in other vascular beds. Brain endothelium contains approximately four times as many mitochondria as found in other capillary endothelial cells. This source of energy is an essential part of the actual barrier, accounting for the rapid degradative process and preventing the penetration of a variety of endogenous and exogenous agents into the CNS. The brain endothelium also contains enzymes specifically involved in the inactivation of neurotransmitters, including monoamine oxidase, cholinesterase, and γ-aminobutyric acid transaminase.

How do substances get into the CNS? Specific carrier-mediated transport processes are present in brain endothelial cells that account for the uptake of a variety of agents into the CNS. It is important to point out that the blood–brain barrier also poses a barrier for substances exiting the CNS. Here again non-lipid-soluble molecules have to pass through the endothelium to exit the brain. Transport systems are also present to remove degradative products and potentially toxic compounds from the CNS.

> The function of the blood–brain barrier is to protect the brain from both endogenous and exogenous substances present in blood that may interfere with neuronal transmission.

Understanding the properties of the different transport systems has permitted specific drugs to be developed that do not penetrate the blood–brain barrier and that act exclusively within the periphery. Examples of this are drugs that are used for the treatment of Parkinson disease. The symptoms of Parkinson disease result from degeneration of the dopaminergic neurons in the substantia nigra leading to deficient dopamine release in the striatum. Therapy includes replacement of dopamine using the precursor L-dopa, which is readily transported into brain. In the periphery, L-dopa can be metabolically inactivated by the enzymes amino acid decarboxylase and catecholamine-O-methyltransferase. To achieve quantities of L-dopa adequate for therapy normally requires administering relatively high levels of the dopamine precursor, which often produces serious and annoying side effects. To minimize these side effects and to optimize the therapeutic dose required to alleviate the symptoms of the disease, selective inhibitors of amino acid decarboxylase and catecholamine-O-methyltransferase are coadministered along with L-dopa. These inhibitors (carbidopa and entecapone, respectively) do not cross the blood–brain barrier and, thus, selectively inhibit these enzymes only in the periphery. Thus, lower doses of L-dopa can be employed to minimize peripheral side effects of this agent.

Specific Transport Mechanisms

Passive Diffusion As previously noted, the blood–brain barrier is a lipid-permeable barrier permitting the passive and facile transport of highly lipid-soluble compounds into the CNS. In the absence of endothelial degradation, the more lipid soluble a substance, the more rapidly it can penetrate the barrier.

> Substances that enter the brain by *passive diffusion* are limited by blood flow.

For example, the barbiturates thiopental and pentobarbital, although structurally similar, differ in their oil/water partition coefficients by a factor of approximately 14-fold. Intravenous injection of thiopental (15 mg/kg) can induce total anesthesia in rats within 30 sec, whereas pentobarbital induces only heavy sedation that occurs between 2 and 4 min after injection. These results can be explained by differences in brain levels of the two barbiturates, with higher brain levels being achieved more rapidly with the more lipid-soluble agent, thiopental, than that with pentobarbital.

Water and gases also readily diffuse across brain capillaries. The half-life for the exchange of brain water varies between 12 and 25 sec and is, to a large extent, limited by cerebral blood flow.

Carrier-Mediated Transport

> Transport mechanisms for *glucose* are highly enriched and stereospecific in brain capillaries.

Transport of glucose is normally in excess of utilization in the CNS. However, under conditions of profound anoxia, such as during a seizure or fasting, uptake may become limiting. The *hexoses,* maltose and mannitol, are also rapidly transported in brain endothelium, whereas galactose is slowly taken up into brain.

> At least three distinct Na^+-dependent transport systems are present in brain capillaries for *amino acids,* one for neutral, one for basic, and one for acidic amino acids.

Essential amino acids that are not synthesized in brain, but are required for neurotransmitter synthesis, are readily transported, whereas amino acids that are formed in brain (e.g., γ-aminobutyric acid) are slowly transported but are avidly removed from the brain. Amino acids of similar structure actually compete for their respective transport systems and can modulate the rate and extent of each other's entry into the CNS.

Monocarboxylic acids such as pyruvate, lactate, and acetate are transported into the brain by separate stereospecific uptake processes.

Purines such as adenine and its nucleoside derivative, adenosine, are readily transported across the blood–brain barrier. In contrast, the pyrimidines are not transported.

Transport of *choline* across brain capillaries may be rate limiting in terms of its utilization in brain. Because it is not synthesized in brain, transport has been proposed to regulate the synthesis of acetylcholine in the CNS. Choline transport is effectively inhibited by tertiary and quaternary amines such as dimethyl-aminoethanol and tetraethylammonium chloride, respectively.

Vitamins are transported into brain by distinct transport systems. The capacity of these systems is low because only small amounts of vitamins are actually utilized.

Efflux Transport

A variety of transport mechanisms are present that account for the efflux of substances out of the CNS. Transport of substances out of the brain occurs possibly by active transport, for example, 5-hydroxyindoleacetic acid, homovanillic acid, and 3-methoxy-4-hydroxyphenylglycol-SO_4.

Areas of Blood–Brain Barrier Breakdown

There are several areas in the brain in which there is a breakdown of the blood–brain barrier, permitting the direct sampling of components in blood.

1. Area protremo—the vomiting center
2. Median eminence of the hypothalamus—controls body metabolism
3. Choroid plexus—there are no tight junctions in the endothelium; the blood–cerebrospinal fluid barrier is produced by tight junctions within the epithelium
4. Pineal gland—production of the hormone melatonin
5. Olfactory bulb—direct uptake (retrograde transport) of substances into the CNS.

STRUCTURE AND FUNCTION OF THE SYNAPSE

> To function efficiently after release from the presynaptic nerve terminal, neurotransmitters must diffuse to the postsynaptic membrane where they bind to their appropriate receptor.

The distance transversed by the neurotransmitters has to be small for the signaling process to work efficiently and effectively. The space between the presynaptic and postsynaptic membranes, the synaptic cleft, is approximately 150–200 Å, allowing for the rapid and proficient propagation of the neurotransmitter signal.

> The presynaptic nerve terminal is the functional site at which small molecule neurotransmitters such as the biogenic amines and amino acids are synthesized. In contrast, the neuropeptides are primarily synthesized in the perikaryon and then subsequently transported down the axon to the nerve terminal.

For the small molecule neurotransmitters, the nerve terminal contains all the enzymes necessary for their synthesis and degradation. Because of the rapid turnover of these neurotransmitters, the presynaptic nerve endings have a very large metabolic capacity. Consistent with this are studies demonstrating the presence of abundant but smaller than normal mitochondria in the nerve terminals.

Neurotransmitters are specifically packaged within storage vesicles within the nerve terminals.

> The function of the storage vesicle is to bind, store, and prevent degradation of the neurotransmitters.

These storage vesicles may contain more than one neurotransmitter or neuromodulator, all of which are released into the synaptic cleft on nerve stimulation. Enzymes may also be present in these vesicles that play a role in the synthesis of neurotransmitters. For example, the enzyme dopamine-β-hydroxylase, which converts dopamine to norepinephrine, is present in the storage vesicles within noradrenergic nerve terminals. Drugs have been designed that function by inhibiting the packaging or binding of neurotransmitters within these vesicles.

In addition to synthesis and storage of the neurotransmitters, the nerve terminal also plays a major role in their metabolism and inactivation.

Degradative enzymes for neurotransmitters and neuromodulators are present in the presynaptic nerve endings. For example, cholinergic nerve terminals contain acetylcholinesterase, which is released into the synaptic cleft to inactivate the released neurotransmitter. Catecholamine-specific nerve terminals contain the outer mitochondrial enzyme, monoamine oxidase, which deaminates and inactivates these neurotransmitters. In addition to enzymatic inactivation of the neurotransmitters, other mechanisms also prevail in the nerve terminals that account for the rapid and efficient termination of neurotransmitter activity. The biogenic amine neurotransmitters, dopamine, norepinephrine, epinephrine, and 5-hydroxytryptamine, are all removed from the synaptic cleft by a high-affinity active reuptake process that rapidly and selectively transports these transmitters back into the nerve terminal. Once inside the nerve terminal, the biogenic amines are either repackaged into storage vesicles or are ultimately inactivated by the enzyme monoamine oxidase, as previously noted.

A more extensive discussion of the properties and function of the synapse is presented in Chapter 4.

NEUROTRANSMITTERS AND NEUROMODULATORS

Neurotransmitters function either by depolarizing or hyperpolarizing the postsynaptic membrane and thus promote or suppress signal propagation, respectively.

However, neurotransmitters can possess both excitatory and inhibitory properties, depending on the specific neuronal connection specified. Below are some endogenous neurotransmitters and their known functional properties.

Biogenic Amines

Biogenic amines (catechol and indole amines) are analogs of phenylethylamine or indole amine. They can be either *excitatory* or *inhibitory*:

1. Dopamine
2. Norepinephrine
3. Epinephrine
4. 5-Hydroxytryptamine
5. Others—neuromodulators, for example, phenylethylamine (α-methylphenylethylamine = amphetamine), tyramine, octopamine (acts as a neurotransmitter in lobster), and tryptamine.

Biogenic amines have numerous functions.

Dopamine (DA) plays a role in movement and behavioral disorders:

1. Parkinson disease—degeneration of dopaminergic neurons in the substantia nigra causing a decrease in dopamine release in the striatum.
2. Schizophrenia (mesolimbic area of the brain)—increased DA receptors, antipsychotic drugs function by blocking dopamine D_2 receptors.
3. Tourette syndrome—dopamine reuptake deficit.

Norepinephrine (NE) plays a role in depression.

A deficiency of norepinephrine in the CNS is related to depression, and inhibitors of norepinephrine neuronal reuptake are antidepressants.

5-Hydroxytryptamine (5-HT, serotonin) plays a role in the following:

1. Depression—a deficiency of 5-HT in the CNS is related to depression [selective serotonin reuptake inhibitors (SSRI) are antidepressants].
2. Actions of LSD—block 5-HT presynaptic receptors in the Raphe nucleus.
3. Others—schizophrenia and migraine headaches.

Acetylcholine

Acetylcholine, which is *excitatory,* is associated with regulating movement in the periphery (neuromuscular junction) and with behavior in the CNS.

There is a decrease of acetylcholine in the cerebral cortex and the hippo-campus in Alzheimer disease and a decrease in the synthesizing enzyme, choline acetyltransferase.

Amino Acids

γ-*Aminobutyric acid* (GABA) is the most prevalent *inhibitory* neurotrans-mitter in the CNS.

A decrease of GABA can lead to convulsions. Benzodiazepines are used for treatment of epilepsy and function by decreasing the K_D for GABA binding to $GABA_A$ receptors. A function has been proposed for GABA in neurological and psychological disorders including Huntington disease, tardive dyskinesia, schiz-ophrenia, anxiety, and Parkinson disease. Other amino acid inhibitory neuro-transmitters (also neuromodulators) include glycine, taurine, and β-alanine.

Glutamate is a major *excitatory* neurotransmitter; during stroke or other brain injury large quantities are released, causing extensive and prolonged neu-ronal damage. N-Methyl-D-aspartate (NMDA) receptors function by regulating Ca^{2+} and Na^+ channels.

Purinergic

Adenosine is among a group of specific receptors found in the hippocampus; it increases cyclic adenosine monophosphate (cAMP) and adenyl cyclase activ-ity. Adenosine triphosphate (ATP) can act as both a neurotransmitter or neuro-modulator.

Peptides

There are many different peptides, for example,

$$SO_4$$

Cholecystokinin	Asp-Tyr-Met-Gly-Trp-Met-Asp-Phe
Enkephalin	Tyr-Gly-Gly-Phe-Leu or –Met

Peptides can act as either neurotransmitters or neuromodulators. They are often packaged and released from storage vesicles into the synaptic cleft along with other small molecule neurotransmitters; for example, NE and DA vesicles often contain cholecystokinin (CCK), and GABA is sometimes coreleased with CCK, somatostatin, or neuropeptide Y.

BIOCHEMISTRY OF BIOGENIC AMINES
Catecholamine Synthesis

> The *catecholamine neurotransmitters* play a major role in regulating a variety of processes in both the peripheral and central nervous systems.

They are synthesized in the brain, sympathetic neurons, and chromaffin cells. In the neuron, synthesis of the three catecholamine neurotransmitters, dopamine, norepinephrine, and epinephrine, occurs primarily in the presynaptic nerve terminal. The biosynthetic pathway, starting from the amino acid precursor phenylalanine, is shown in Figure 5–1.

Tyrosine Hydroxylase

> The synthesis of the catecholamines begins with the enzyme *tyrosine hydroxylase.*

The substrate for the enzyme, tyrosine, is readily transported into the CNS across the blood–brain barrier. Only about 2% of the tyrosine that enters the CNS is actually converted to catecholamine neurotransmitters. The reaction proceeds via a ping-pong mechanism requiring the pteridine cofactor, tetrahydrobiopterin. The enzyme is found exclusively in the catecholamine terminal and is present as both a membrane-bound and soluble enzyme species.

Tyrosine hydroxylase is considered to be the rate-limiting enzyme for synthesis of the catecholamines because its overall activity is approximately 100–1000 times lower than that of the other enzymes in the biosynthetic pathway, and under physiological conditions the two substrates, tyrosine and tetrahydrobiopterin, are probably not saturating. Tyrosine hydroxylase activity can be regulated transcriptionally and posttranscriptionally by phosphorylation and end-product inhibition. A variety of stimuli including stress, electrical stimulation, and drugs promote the rapid phosphorylation of tyrosine hydroxylase. Phosphorylation regulates the properties of the hydroxylase by changing the kinetic

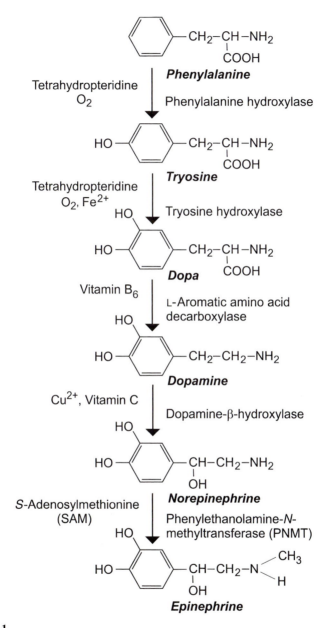

Figure 5–1
Synthesis of catecholamine neurotransmitters: dopamine, norepinephrine, and epinephrine.

characteristics of the enzyme. The K_m for tetrahydrobiopterin binding is decreased approximately threefold, from 200 to 88 µM, and there is a 30% increase in the V_{max}. In addition the K_i for binding of the end-product inhibitor, norepinephrine, is increased almost eightfold, from 6 to 45 µM. A variety of kinases are responsible for this phosphorylation including cAMP-dependent protein kinase A (PKA) and CAM kinase. Phosphorylation of tyrosine hydroxylase, which increases enzyme activity, is considered to be important in the short-term regulation of the enzyme activity. In contrast, increased transcription of the gene for tyrosine hydroxylase, induced by a variety of factors, is generally considered important for the long-term maintenance of overall enzyme activity.

L-Aromatic Amino Acid Decarboxylase

> The second enzyme in the pathway for synthesis of the catecholamines is L-aromatic amino acid decarboxylase.

Although sometimes referred to as dopa decarboxylase in the literature, this latter name is really a misnomer as it implies preferential binding for the amino acid L-dopa to the enzyme. In fact, this enzyme is rather nonselective and is actually capable of decarboxylating a variety of aromatic amino acids. It utilizes pyridoxal phosphate as a cofactor, and its activity greatly exceeds that of tyrosine hydroxylase in the catecholamine nerve terminal. However, unlike tyrosine hydroxylase, this decarboxylase is not selectively present only in nerve terminals.

Dopamine β-Hydroxylase

> Dopamine β-hydroxylase is responsible for the conversion of dopamine into norepinephrine and thus is not present in dopaminergic nerve terminals.

Dopamine β-hydroxylase is a glycoprotein containing two to four residues of Cu^{2+} per molecule of enzyme. It requires molecular oxygen and ascorbic acid for activity. There is both a membrane-bound and soluble form of the enzyme. Approximately 90% of the enzyme in the nerve terminal is membrane bound and resides within the catecholamine storage vesicles. In the perikarya, the ratio of the two species is approximately 50:50. The enzyme is relatively nonspecific in that any of the phenylethylamine derivatives, including phenylethylamine and tyramine, can also be readily hydroxylated. Because it is located in the storage vesicles, the enzyme is released into the synaptic cleft on exocytosis.

Phenylethanolamine *N*-Methyltransferase

Phenylethanolamine N-methyltransferase (PNMT) is a soluble enzyme responsible for the conversion of norepinephrine to epinephrine.

PNMT utilizes *S*-adenosylmethionine as the methyl donator and is located in synaptic endings. It is transcriptionally regulated by corticosteroids, which increase expression of the gene. Thus, steroids have the potential to influence norepinephrine concentrations in both the periphery and CNS by regulating PNMT synthesis.

Inactivation of Catecholamine Neurotransmitters

Reuptake of Catecholamines

The major route by which the catecholamine neurotransmitters are functionally inactivated is by active *reuptake* back into the presynaptic nerve terminal.

Reuptake into presynaptic nerve terminals is referred to as *uptake I* and is characterized by a saturable, stereospecific, high-affinity transport system. In contrast, uptake into glia and other cells is classified as *uptake II* and is characterized by a low-affinity transport carrier system. Uptake I requires a non-esterified *m*- or *p*-OH on the aromatic ring for transport, and therefore the *O*-methylated products (COMT products, see below) are not transported back into the nerve terminal. Transport of the catecholamines is energy dependent and, thus, temperature, pH, and ouabain sensitive. Selective inhibitors of uptake I (tricyclic antidepressants, etc.) are used in the treatment of depression.

Catecholamine Degradative Enzymes Although reuptake of the catecholamines is responsible for the functional removal and inactivation of these substances from the synaptic cleft, their enzymatic degradation occurs within both the nerve terminal and surrounding astrocytes.

Three enzymes are responsible for the catabolism of the catecholamines: *monoamine oxidase, catechol-O-methyltransferase,* and *phenolsulfotransferase.*

Figure 5–2 illustrates the cellular localization of both the biosynthetic and catecholamine degradative enzymes in the CNS.

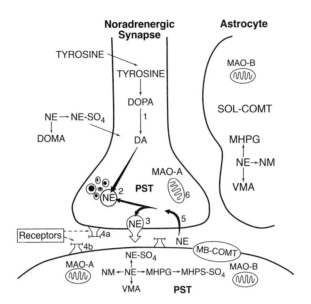

Figure 5–2

Biochemical processes regulating the noradrenergic nerve terminal. (1) Tyrosine hydroxylase—the rate-limiting step for synthesis of the catecholamines, regulated by phosphorylation and transcription. (2) Norepinephrine (NE) storage vesicles—contain dopamine-β-hydroxylase, ATP, and other proteins, often packaged with other peptide neurotransmitters. (3) Release of norepinephrine—stimulated by Ca^{2+} and stimulated by amphetamine and other sympathomimetic amines. (4) Receptors for norepinephrine—specific presynaptic (4a) and postsynaptic (4b) receptors regulate norepinephrine synthesis and action, respectively. (5) Uptake I—active mechanism for reuptake of norepinephrine into presynaptic nerve terminals; inhibitors act as antidepressants. (6) Monoamine oxidase (MAO)—the A form of monoamine oxidase present in neurons resides in the outer mitochondrial membrane; inhibitors of MAO are antidepressants. SOL-COMT, soluble form of COMT; MB-COMT, membrane-bound form of COMT; PST, phenol sulfotransferase; DA, domamine; NM, normetanephrine; MHPG, 3-methoxy-4-hydroxyphenylglycol; VMA, vanillylmandelic acid.

> *Monoamine oxidase* (MAO) is the major enzyme responsible for degradation of the catecholamine neurotransmitters.

Two forms of the enzyme have been isolated and both map to the X chromosome. The *A form,* which deaminates dopamine, norepinephrine, and 5-hydroxytryptamine, is selectively localized in neurons. The *B form,* which deaminates dopamine, norepinephrine, and phenylethylamine, selectively resides in astrocytes, although some serotonergic neurons also appear to contain this form of the oxidase. Both forms of MAO are localized in the outer mitochondrial membrane and contain covalently bound flavin adenine dinucleotide (FAD) as the cofactor. The reaction requires oxygen and kinetically proceeds via a ping-pong-like reaction mechanism. Selective inhibitors of MAO A and B have been developed. Inhibitors of the A form act as antidepressants, whereas inhibitors of the B form are used in the treatment of Parkinson disease. MAO is generally considered to be in huge excess in the CNS, and approximately 80% inhibition of the total enzymatic activity by the MAO inhibitors is required to achieve a therapeutic response.

As illustrated in Figure 5–3, the aldehyde formed from deamination of the biogenic amines by MAO can subsequently be oxidized by aldehyde dehydrogenase to the corresponding carboxylic acid or reduced to the alcohol by the actions of aldehyde reductase. Oxidation to the acid occurs preferentially in the periphery, whereas reduction of the norepinephrine deaminated metabolite, 3,4-dihydroxyphenylacetaldehyde, is preferentially reduced in the CNS to the glycol product, 3,4-dihydroxyphenylethyleneglycol.

> Catechol-O-methyltransferase (COMT) is present in the CNS as both a membrane-bound and a soluble enzyme.

Both forms of the enzyme are derived from the same gene, with the membrane-bound species possessing a hydrophobic tail on the 3′-end, which is responsible for its attachment to membranes. Differences in the posttranslational processing of the gene product are responsible for the presence of the two species. The membrane-bound form, which may be neuronal, has a higher affinity but lower V_{max} for the catecholamines than the soluble enzyme, which predominates exclusively in astrocytes. The soluble form is generally considered to be the major form of COMT primarily because it possesses the higher V_{max} and, thus, has a greater capacity to methylate catecholamines. However, at physiological concentrations of the catecholamines, the membrane-bound form in human brain may be the more active of the two species. Both forms of COMT utilize S-adenosylmethionine as the methyl donor and both have a very broad substrate specificity exemplified by their ability to methylate essentially any catechol substrate. Selective peripheral inhibitors of COMT, which do not penetrate the blood–brain barrier, have been developed for the treatment of Parkinson disease.

As illustrated in Figure 5–3, both the catecholamine and its deaminated products undergo methylation by COMT. The 3′-methylated product is the major metabolite formed, although the 4′ product is also produced in vivo. Methylation of either hydroxyl group results in inactivation of these neurotransmitters.

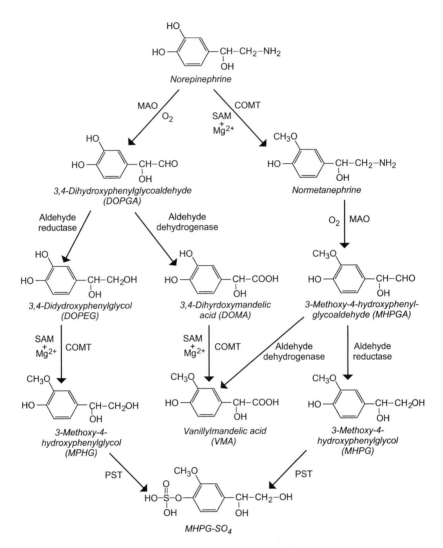

Figure 5–3
Metabolism of norepinephrine.

Phenolsulfotransferase (PST) (Figure 5–4), although not regarded as a major enzyme responsible for the inactivation of the catecholamine neurotransmitters, nevertheless possesses the highest affinity (K_m approximately 1 µM) of any of the enzymes for these neurologically active agents. Multiple forms of PST have been identified in human brain and all are selectively located in neurons. The M-form

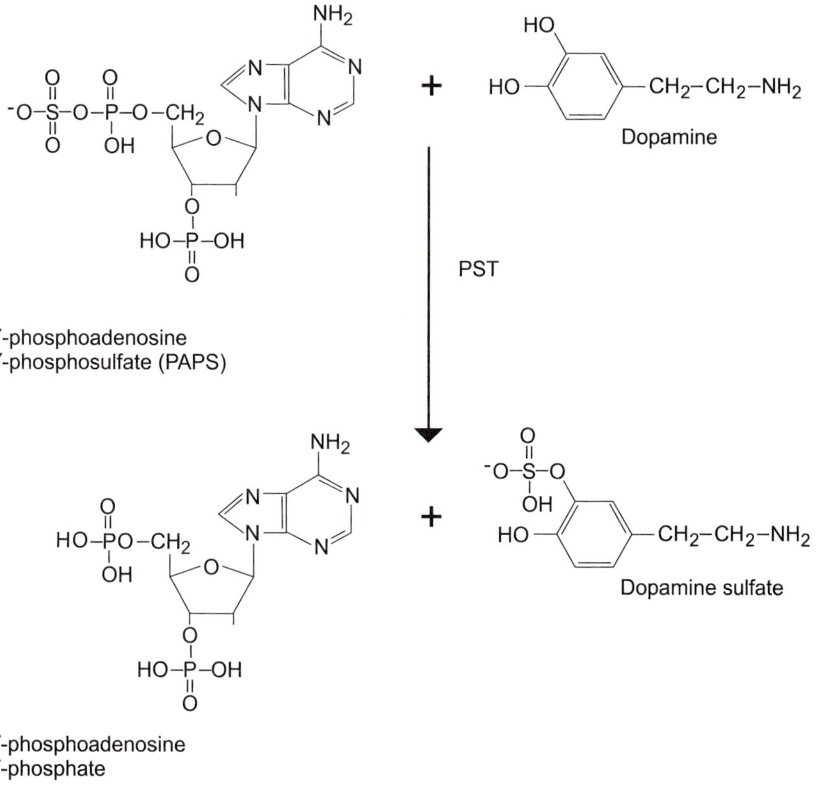

Figure 5–4
Reaction catalyzed by phenolsulfotransferase.

of PST (STM) selectively sulfates the catecholamine neurotransmitters. It utilizes 3'-phosphoadenosine-5'-phosphosulfate as the sulfate donor. The role and contribution of PST in the inactivation of the catecholamine neurotransmitters are not fully understood.

5-Hydroxytryptamine Synthesis

The indole amine, *5-hydroxytryptamine* (5-HT), is an important neurotransmitter involved in the regulation of a variety of behavioral and peripheral disorders.

Like the catecholamines, 5-HT synthesis occurs primarily within the serotonergic presynaptic nerve endings in the brain. 5-HT is bound to a specific binding protein within storage vesicles and is released on exocytosis. Only 1–2% of the total 5-HT in the body is actually found within the CNS. The biosynthetic pathway for 5-HT is illustrated in Figure 5–5.

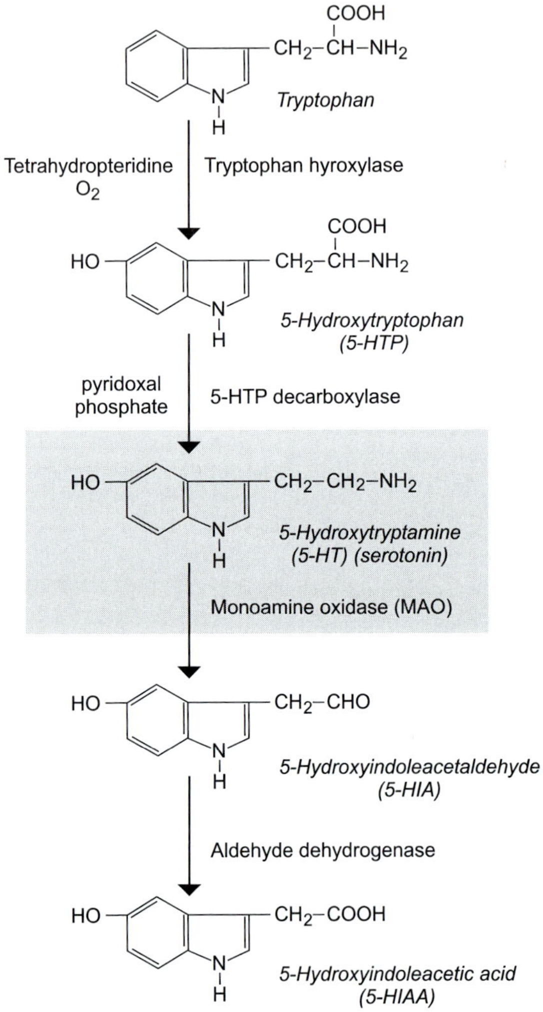

Figure 5–5
Synthesis and degradation of 5-hydroxytryptamine.

Tryptophan Hydroxylase

> The function of *tryptophan hydroxylase* is similar to that of tyrosine hydroxylase in that it may be the rate-limiting step for synthesis of 5-HT.

Like tyrosine hydroxylase, tryptophan hydroxylase also utilizes tetrahydrobiopterin as a cofactor. At physiological concentration, the enzyme is not saturated with tryptophan or tetrahydrobiopterin and transport of this amino acid into the CNS is probably rate limiting for production of 5-HT. Tryptophan hydroxylase activity is regulated at the level of transcription and not at the level of end-product inhibition. The enzyme can also be activated and phosphorylated on Ser-58 by PKA.

L-Aromatic Amino Acid Decarboxylase   The form of L-aromatic amino acid decarboxylase that decarboxylates 5-HT is located in 5-HT nerve endings. It has recently been cloned and has been shown to be identical to the form of the enzyme responsible for the decarboxylation of L-dopa.

5-Hydroxytryptamine Inactivation

5-HT Neuronal Reuptake

> Similar to the catecholamine neurotransmitters, *reuptake of 5-HT* into serotonergic presynaptic nerve terminals is the major route for synaptic inactivation.

The 5-HT membrane carrier is a high-affinity, sodium-dependent transporter and possesses approximately 50% homology with that of the norepinephrine and dopamine transporters. Selective inhibitors of 5-HT reuptake (chlorimipramine, paroxetine, sertraline, and fluoxetine) are currently used as antidepressants and are used for the treatment of obsessive-compulsive disorder.

5-Hydroxytryptamine Degradative Enzymes

> The major pathway for 5-HT degradation (Figure 5–6) is via deamination by the A form of *MAO,* which is selectively located in presynaptic nerve endings.

Selective inhibition of the A form of MAO is believed to be responsible for the antidepressant actions of the monoamine oxidase inhibitors (MAOIs). Currently,

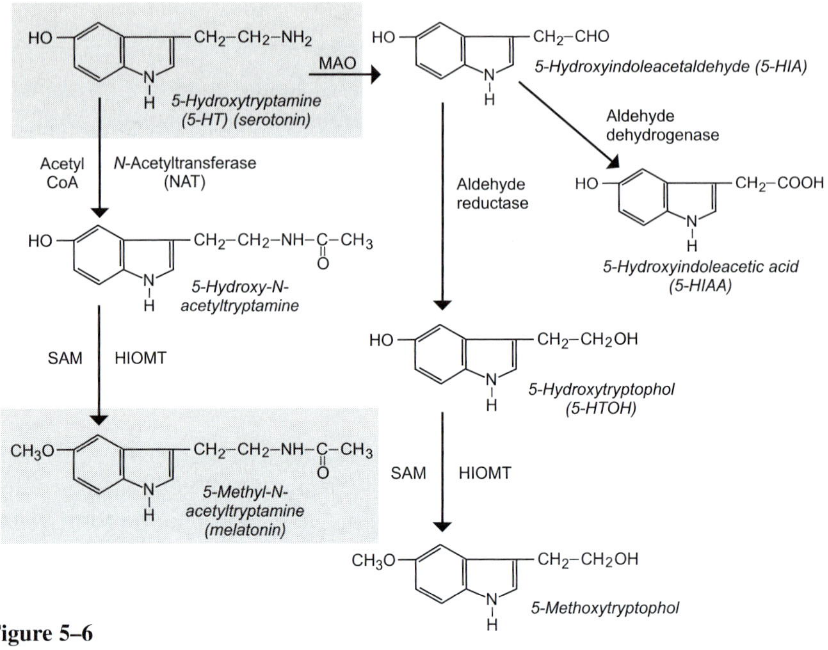

Figure 5–6
Metabolites and other biosynthetic reactions of 5-hydroxytryptamine.

the MAOIs used clinically irreversibly inhibit the oxidase and are relatively non-specific in that they inhibit both forms of MAO equally. New highly selective reversible MAO A inhibitors are currently being tested for treatment of depression.

Other Reactions

5-HT is also the precursor for the pineal hormone melatonin.

To form melatonin, 5-HT is initially acetylated by the enzyme N-acetyl-transferase, and subsequently methylated by indole amine-O-methyltransferase. Acetylation by N-acetyltransferase is the rate-limiting step for synthesis of melatonin production, and its expression is elevated by cAMP and down-regulated by light. Daily circadian rhythms persist for melatonin even in the absence of a light stimulus, as the levels of N-acetyltransferase are regulated by the circadian pattern produced within the suprachiasmatic nuclei of the brain.

During the past several years, there has been an increased awareness of the potential role of melatonin in regulating a variety of physiological, pathophysiological, and neuroendocrine processes. Melatonin is known to influence a variety of physiological processes including hypothalamic control of circadian rhythms, regulation of temperature, sexual maturation, and immune system activity as well as regulation of reproductive function in seasonally breeding animals.

At least three high-affinity cell surface receptors for melatonin have been identified, Mel 1a, Mel 1b, and Mel 1c. Mel 1a and 1b are present in all mammals, whereas the Mel 1c receptor has been identified only in birds. The Mel 1a and 1b receptors display 60% homology, and both contain seven membrane-spanning domains. These transmembrane receptors are linked to the guanine nucleotide Gi and suppress adenylate cyclase activity. In addition, melatonin, at high pharmacological concentrations, is a very potent free-radical scavenger capable of preventing oxidative stress in a number of biological systems. Its interaction with highly reactive oxygen species within the cell is facilitated by the fact that melatonin is lipid soluble and readily crosses the plasma membrane.

SYNTHESIS AND DEGRADATION OF ACETYLCHOLINE

The role of acetylcholine as a neurotransmitter has been known since the early part of the twentieth century. Its physiological function and the biochemical systems involved in its regulation have been extensively studied. Neurotoxins used in World War I and even in the present are potent inhibitors of acetylcholine function. There is strong evidence in the literature that a number of disease states are linked to cholinergic dysfunction.

> Myasthenia gravis syndrome, Huntington disease, Alzheimer disease, familial dysautonomia, and Lambert-Eaton myasthenic syndrome are all associated with impaired acetylcholine function.

Synthesis and Storage of Acetylcholine

> The biological machinery necessary for the synthesis (Figure 5–7) and degradation of *acetylcholine* is present in the cholinergic presynaptic nerve terminals. The enzyme involved in synthesis of this neurotransmitter is *choline acetyltransferase.*

Choline acetyltransferase resides both within the cytosolic and synaptic membrane vesicles of the nerve terminal. Although the majority of the transferase is present in the cytosol, the membrane-bound form displays the highest specific activity and may be the more physiologically relevant form in vivo.

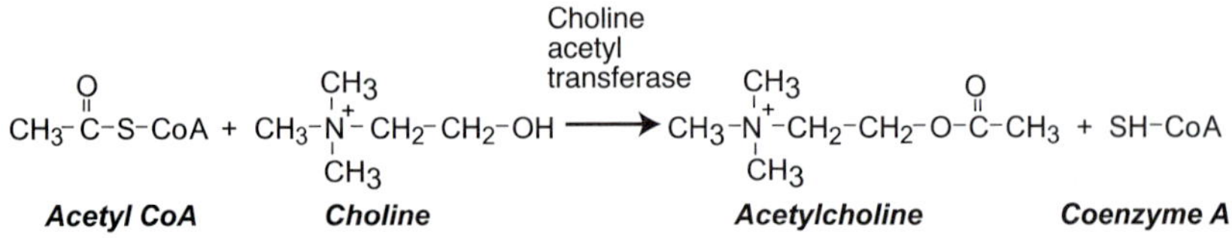

$$CH_3\text{-}\overset{O}{\overset{\|}{C}}\text{-S-CoA} + CH_3\text{-}\overset{CH_3}{\underset{CH_3}{\overset{|}{N^+}}}\text{-}CH_2\text{-}CH_2\text{-OH} \xrightarrow{\text{Choline acetyl transferase}} CH_3\text{-}\overset{CH_3}{\underset{CH_3}{\overset{|}{N^+}}}\text{-}CH_2\text{-}CH_2\text{-O-}\overset{O}{\overset{\|}{C}}\text{-}CH_3 + SH\text{-CoA}$$

Acetyl CoA　　　　　　*Choline*　　　　　　　　　*Acetylcholine*　　　　　*Coenzyme A*

Figure 5–7
Biosynthesis of acetylcholine.

Acetylcholine formed in the synaptic nerve endings is packaged and stored in vesicles that are released on exocytosis. Newly synthesized acetylcholine appears to be preferentially released on nerve stimulation. Acetylcholine synthesized in the nerve terminal is transported into the storage vesicles by a specific transport carrier whose gene is located within an intron of the choline acetyltransferase gene. This implies a coregulation between synthesis and storage of this neurotransmitter.

The affinity of choline for choline acetyltransferase is rather low, possessing a K_m of almost 1 mM. Thus, under physiological conditions, the enzyme is normally not saturated in the CNS. Accordingly, choline levels are thought to be limiting and enzyme activity is presumed to be regulated by transport of choline into the CNS. High-affinity transport of choline in the CNS is specific for acetylcholine nerve terminals, and approximately 50–80% of what is transported is utilized for acetylcholine synthesis. Other than the choline that is transported into the brain, the major source of choline in the neuron is from hydrolysis of phosphatidylcholine. Feedback product inhibition by acetylcholine may also regulate choline acetyltransferase activity in brain.

Degradation of Acetylcholine

Unlike the biogenic amine neurotransmitters that are functionally inactivated within the synaptic cleft by an active neuronal reuptake process, acetylcholine is poorly transported across the presynaptic nerve membrane by a low-affinity transporter.

Acetylcholine is therefore primarily inactivated either by simple diffusion or degradation by acetylcholinesterase within the synaptic cleft itself (Figure 5–8).

It is estimated that acetylcholine released into the cleft is degraded within 2 msec. The cholinesterases responsible for hydrolyzing acetylcholine are subdivided into two categories, acetylcholinesterase and butyryl- or pseudocholinesterase. Because of its higher activity and specificity, acetylcholinesterase is probably the

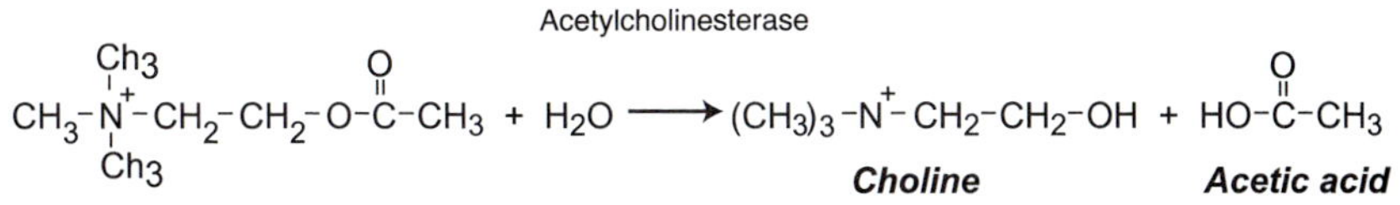

$$CH_3-\underset{\underset{CH_3}{|}}{\overset{\overset{CH_3}{|}}{N^+}}-CH_2-CH_2-O-\overset{\overset{O}{\|}}{C}-CH_3 + H_2O \xrightarrow{\text{Acetylcholinesterase}} (CH_3)_3-N^+-CH_2-CH_2-OH + HO-\overset{\overset{O}{\|}}{C}-CH_3$$

$\textbf{\textit{Choline}}$ $\textbf{\textit{Acetic acid}}$

Figure 5–8
Degradation of acetylcholine.

functionally active esterase within the nervous system in humans. Multiple forms of acetylcholinesterase, differing in their solubility, mode of membrane attachment, and tertiary structure, are present within the nerve terminal. Studies have demonstrated that multiple forms of this enzyme arise from alternative processing of messenger RNA from a single gene.

Choline that is formed within the synaptic cleft after hydrolysis of acetylcholine is transported back into the nerve terminal and is reutilized to make acetylcholine. Conservation of choline is important as it is probably limiting for acetylcholine synthesis, and approximately 50% of the choline that is formed is taken back into the neuron.

SYNTHESIS AND DEGRADATION OF γ-AMINOBUTYRIC ACID (GABA)

GABA is by far the most prevalent inhibitory neurotransmitter in the CNS, being present in millimolar concentrations. As noted previously, it has been proposed that it functions in a variety of neurological and psychological disorders including Huntington disease, alcoholism, tardive dyskinesia, schizophrenia, anxiety, and Parkinson disease. Being a major inhibitory neurotransmitter, xenobiotics that interfere with GABA synthesis have been shown to induce convulsions in humans.

GABA Synthesis

> GABA is formed within the brain by a metabolic pathway classified as the GABA shunt.

GABA is a charged molecule at physiological pH and does not penetrate the blood–brain barrier. Therefore, it must be formed within the brain by de novo synthesis via the decarboxylation of glutamate. This is accomplished by glutamic acid decarboxylase (GAD), an enzyme found exclusively in GABAminergic nerve terminals. As illustrated in Figure 5–9, glutamic acid is produced by the

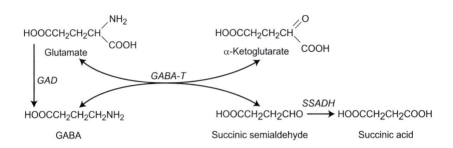

Figure 5–9
Synthesis and metabolism of GABA.

actions of GABA α-oxogluterate transaminase, an enzyme that converts α-ketogluterate, formed in the Krebs cycle, to glutamic acid. The GABA that is produced is then converted to succinic semialdehyde, which can reenter the Krebs cycle by its metabolism to succinic acid by the enzyme succinic semialdehyde dehydrogenase.

Two related genes for GAD have been identified in the CNS, and both are only approximately 50% saturated with the cofactor pyridoxal phosphate, implying that GAD activity is regulated by the availability of its cofactor. Consistent with this is the observation that deficiencies of vitamin B_6 have been shown to cause convulsions in infants.

GABA Degradation

> The actions of GABA in the synapse are, most likely, terminated by its transport back into the nerve ending or the surrounding astrocytes by a sodium-dependent process.

This is presumed to be the major inactivating mechanism, but this hypothesis results from the lack of any other known mechanism that can account for GABA degradation in the synaptic cleft. After it is taken up into the nerve terminal or astrocytes, the principal enzyme responsible for GABA inactivation is *GABA transaminase* (GABA-T). This enzyme, which is associated with mitochondria, converts GABA to succinic semialdehyde and in the process donates the amine group to α-ketoglutaric acid to re-form glutamate. Like GAD, GABA-T also utilizes pyridoxal phosphate as a cofactor. However, unlike GAD, the enzyme is saturated with the cofactor and is found extensively outside the CNS. Enzyme activity is not regulated by pyridoxal phosphate levels but is probably controlled by α-ketogluterate levels. Within the CNS, the majority of GABA-T is associated with nonneuronal mitochondria, suggesting that it may be preferentially located in astrocytes. This implies that GABA, which is taken back up into the presynaptic nerve terminal, is preferentially reutilized, whereas GABA that is transported into glia is converted to succinic semialdehyde, which reenters the Krebs cycle and eventually ends up as glutamate. The glutamate formed within the glia is metabolized to glutamine by the manganese-dependent enzyme glutamine synthetase, which is selectively localized to astroglia in the CNS. The glutamine produced in these glial cells is then available for transport back into neurons.

> Two receptors for GABA have been identified: $GABA_A$ and $GABA_B$.

$GABA_A$ is postsynaptic and is the major inhibitory receptor site in the CNS. It is coupled to the Cl^- channel. Specific sites within this receptor are capable of selectively binding barbiturates, benzodiazepines, and picrotoxin. Barbiturates are presumed to activate the Cl^- channel directly, whereas benzodiazepines bind to an allosteric site resulting in an approximately 10-fold increase in the affinity of GABA for its receptor. In contrast, the $GABA_B$ receptors are heterodimers coupled to G-proteins, causing a decrease in cAMP formation. $GABA_B$ receptors are primarily presynaptic where they decrease Ca^{2+} influx, thereby attenuating neurotransmitter release. There are also postsynaptic, inhibitory $GABA_B$ receptors that open K^+ channels.

SYNTHESIS AND DEGRADATION OF GLUTAMATE

Glutamate, along with aspartate, is found in excessively high levels in the CNS, where it acts as a powerful excitatory neurotransmitter.

> L-Glutamate is synthesized in the nerve terminal from glucose via the Krebs cycle and by transamination of α-oxoglutarate. It is also produced in glial cells by the actions of glutaminase, which converts glutamine to glutamate.

Glutamate is stored in synaptic vesicles in the nerve terminal and is released by a calcium-dependent exocytotic process. The actions of glutamate are terminated by a high-affinity transport system into either the presynaptic nerve endings or into glial cells. There are three distinct glutamate transport systems identified in brain, two of which have been associated with glial uptake of glutamate. Within glial cells, glutamate is converted to glutamine by the enzyme glutamine synthetase. Astrocytic glutamine is subsequently taken back up into the neighboring nerve terminals where it is converted back to glutamate.

Although discussed in greater detail elsewhere in this book, it is necessary to briefly mention that there is considerable interest in the different receptors in brain for glutamate and aspartate.

> Glutamate receptors are divided into *ionotropic receptors,* which contain a channel as part of the receptor protein, and *metabotropic receptors,* which are linked to G-proteins.

There are three types of ionotropic glutamate receptors: N-methyl-D-aspartate (NMDA), 2-(aminomethyl)phenylacetic acid (AMPA), and kainate receptors. The NMDA receptor is of particular interest because it is calcium permeable and voltage dependent. The NMDA receptor must bind both glycine and glutamate before it is activated. As is now clear, excess release of glutamate and/or aspartate can lead to neuronal cell death on binding to these receptors. For example, there is considerable information suggesting that much of the neuronal injury occurring after a stroke is actually caused by the delayed neurotoxic actions of released glutamate.

SYNTHESIS AND DEGRADATION OF GLYCINE

Glycine is not an essential amino acid, but it plays an important role as an inhibitory neurotransmitter or neuromodulator in the CNS.

> The major precursor of *glycine* is serine, which undergoes a reversible folate-dependent reaction catalyzed by the enzyme serine transhydroxymethylase.

The actions of glycine in the synapse are terminated by its reuptake back into the nerve endings via high-affinity transport systems. Two glycine transport proteins have been cloned, one of which is located in neurons and the other in glial cells. Neuronal receptors for glycine have been cloned and appear to belong to the same gene superfamily as the acetylcholine and $GABA_A$ receptors.

NEUROPEPTIDES

Numerous peptides that have been isolated in recent years fulfill, at least in part, the criteria for a neurotransmitter. Physiological as well as functional concentrations of these neuropeptides are two to three orders of magnitude lower than that of the biogenic amines and other small molecule neurotransmitters previously discussed. Also unlike the small molecule neurotransmitters, neuropeptides are synthesized in the soma, which contains the necessary biochemical machinery, including ribosomes and Golgi apparatus, required for formation and posttranslational modification of proteins (Figure 5–10).

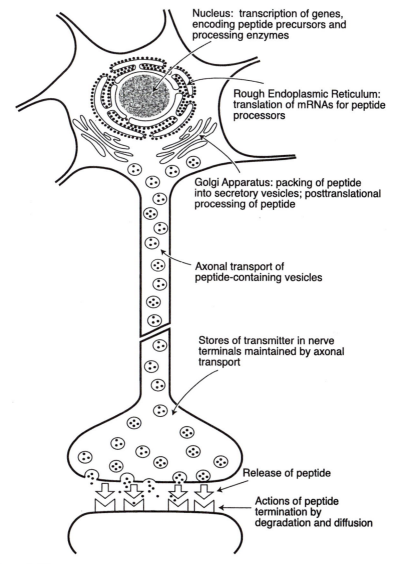

Nucleus: transcription of genes, encoding peptide precursors and processing enzymes

Rough Endoplasmic Reticulum: translation of mRNAs for peptide processors

Golgi Apparatus: packing of peptide into secretory vesicles; posttranslational processing of peptide

Axonal transport of peptide-containing vesicles

Stores of transmitter in nerve terminals maintained by axonal transport

Release of peptide

Actions of peptide termination by degradation and diffusion

Figure 5–10
Neuropeptide synthesis and transport.

Neuropeptides are synthesized on the rough endoplasmic reticulum as inactive precursors referred to as prohormones.

These proteins are packaged in vesicles and transported sequentially to the *cis, medial,* and *trans*-Golgi apparatus, where they undergo posttranslational modification. A variety of structural and chemical changes occur within each compartment of the Golgi apparatus, prerequisites for formation of the fully active neuropeptides. These include proteolysis, glycosylation, phosphorylation, and sulfation. Once processed, the peptides are packaged in vesicles assembled in the trans-Golgi network and transported down the axon to the nerve terminal. Inhibition of axonal transport with antimicrotubual agents such as colchicines results in the accumulation of neuropeptides in the soma. Once transported to the presynaptic nerve terminal, neuropeptides are packaged within synaptic vesicles and released into the synaptic cleft, often along with the classical small molecule neurotransmitters. Peptides are then degraded by a variety of peptidases within the cleft and surrounding fluid.

Release of neuropeptides from the presynaptic nerve ending is similar to that of the small molecule neurotransmitters in that it is Ca^{2+} dependent. There are no reuptake processes to inactivate the released neuropeptides, and reutilization of existing peptide does not occur. Thus, continued synthesis of new peptide is required to maintain levels within the nerve terminal. It is clear that regulation of the functionally active forms of the neuropeptides occurs at all levels, including transcription, translation, and posttranslational modification. Thus, factors that enhance or disrupt any of these steps will alter neuropeptide activity in both the CNS and periphery. Accordingly, disruption of neuropeptide synthesis or axonal transport by neurotoxins can have a profound effect on the function of neurons in the central and peripheral nervous system.

· C H A P T E R · 6 ·

SENSORY SYSTEMS

·

Malcolm Slaughter

Properties of Sensory Receptors

Organization of Sensory Information

Sensory Systems

· · · · · · · · · · · ·

PROPERTIES OF SENSORY RECEPTORS
Transduction

The process of *transduction,* the conversion of energy from one form to another, is the first step in each of the sensory systems.

In each case, external stimuli are transduced into electrical energy, which is the information medium of the nervous system: light energy, sound energy, mechanical energy, or chemical energy is converted to electrical signals in neurons. In each modality, the final result is an electrical potential formed by a specialized detector cell (the receptor cell); the generated voltage is called a receptor

117

potential. This is a graded potential, similar to the excitatory postsynaptic potential (EPSP) formed at a synapse.

Transduction also requires *amplification,* because the energy detected may be very small: a photon of light, a nanometer vibration of sound, or the noncovalent binding energy of an odor molecule. The G-protein system is frequently employed for amplification, as in olfaction, vision, and some forms of gustation. A notable exception is the auditory system, probably because the G-protein system is too slow to follow high-frequency sound waves. The G-protein system in transduction is similar to the metabotropic ligand-gated receptor system (Figure 6–1).

Cyclic Nucleotide–Gated Channels

Many forms of sensory transduction depend on channels that are opened or closed by cyclic nucleotides.

As described below, light-regulated channels in photoreceptors are opened by cyclic guanosine monophosphate (cGMP), and related channels in the olfactory system are opened by cyclic adenosine monophosphate (cAMP). The cyclic nucleotide–gated channel is a six transmembrane protein that is similar in appearance to voltage-gated channels. These channels are regulated by the binding of cyclic nucleotides to the cytoplasmic surface of the channel.

Sensory Decomposition

There is a great variety of information in a sensory signal, and the nervous system usually breaks this information down into subunits and conveys each separately to the brain. This process is called *decomposition.*

For example, the entire spectrum of light is broken down into three colors: red, green, and blue. There are cone photoreceptors for each of these colors, and our final perception of color depends on computing the color of the stimulus based on the relative stimulation of the three types of cones. Video cameras use a similar methodology. Intensity of a signal is conveyed separately, usually with a log scale conversion. For example, bright red light and dim red light are both conveyed by red-sensitive cones, but the former produces a larger receptor potential and the magnitude of that potential is proportional to the log of the brightness.

Another form of signal decomposition is based on rate. Fast signals often carry different information and are carried by different cells. For example, in the

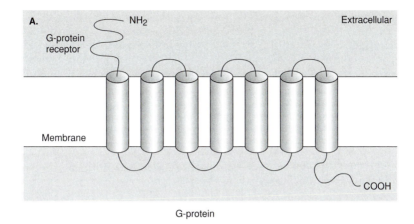

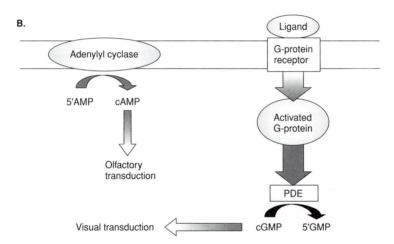

Figure 6–1
(**A**) Seven transmembrane receptor proteins include metabotropic receptors found at the synapse and also proteins involved in transduction of some sensory modalities. (**B**) Receptor binding activates a G-protein, which goes on to activate enzymes such as adenylyl cyclase and phosphodiesterase (PDE). These enzymes regulate levels of second messengers: cAMP and cGMP.

auditory system fast and slow sound waves are detected by different receptors, at opposite ends of the cochlea. In the visual system, cones are able to respond to signals that are too fast for rods. Furthermore, fast signals from cones are conveyed to neurons that are specialized for detection of motion, whereas the slower signals convey color and spatial information.

Adaptation

A property of all sensory systems is *adaptation.* For example, a buzzing noise in a room will be noticeable for only a short time. Sensory systems are designed to detect a stimulus that is significantly different than normal (background). Background can change enormously (compare the level of light on a moonlit night with the level of light on a sunny beach), and receptors are incapable of encoding a full range of stimuli at one time.

> Thus *adaptation* is a mechanism that sets receptors to encode the middle of the range of stimuli likely to be encountered.

We "dark adapt" to the darkness of a movie theatre and then we "light adapt" to daylight after the movie. The adaptation system modifies the transduction system. Weber's law describes our ability to detect a stimulus in the presence of an adapting background; it states that our threshold for detection increases as the background increases: log threshold/log background = constant.

Lateral Inhibition

A common characteristic of sensory systems is lateral inhibition. This often occurs at the first stage of detection, at the receptor cells. Examples are the somatosensory, visual, and olfactory systems.

> In *lateral inhibition,* a signal that stimulates one receptor suppresses surrounding (lateral) receptor cells.

As a result, signals conveyed by the most strongly stimulated receptors are accentuated.

ORGANIZATION OF SENSORY INFORMATION

Topographic Organization

> Sensory signals in the visual and somatosensory systems are *topographically organized,* so that adjacent stimuli in the external world activate adjacent receptors (in the retina or skin), and these receptors send signals to adjacent locations in the brain (the visual or somatosensory cortex).

The auditory system is tonotopically organized, reproducing the tonal (pitch) organization along the length of the basilar membrane. The olfactory system is topographically organized, with different odorants producing different spatial patterns of activity in the olfactory bulb. However, the representation in the cortex is not a perfectly scaled map of the external world. For example, some regions of the retina or skin are greatly enlarged in the cortex. The central area of vision (the fovea) and the skin of the head and hands are sensory regions that have a magnified representation in the cortex.

The Thalamic Relay

> Information from all the sensory systems passes through the *thalamus,* a relay station to the cerebral cortex.

The sensory information for each modality is carried separately in a distinct nucleus within the thalamus. Signals from each thalamic nucleus project to the corresponding primary sensory area of the cortex. The sensory cortex is a well-organized structure consisting of six layers. The thalamic input comes into layers three and four. Columns can be found in an arrangement that is perpendicular to the layers. The stack of neurons in each cortical column relays related information and is distinct from the stack of neurons in adjacent columns. This is best exemplified in the visual system, in which adjacent columns are referred to as ocular dominance columns and receive input from one eye or the other. Within each ocular dominance column, properties such as orientation are arranged stepwise along the column.

SENSORY SYSTEMS

The Visual System

Visual Transduction

> *Transduction* in the *visual system* begins with capture of a photon by a photosensitive pigment.

The best studied pigment is rhodopsin, which is found in rods. When a photon is captured, it provides the energy to change the conformation of the pigment protein molecule. This leads to activation of a G-protein, called transducin, resulting in the activation of the enzyme phosphodiesterase (PDE) (Figure 6–2). This enzyme cleaves cGMP. In darkness, photoreceptors have high levels of cGMP that act as an internal transmitter to promote the opening of cation-permeable

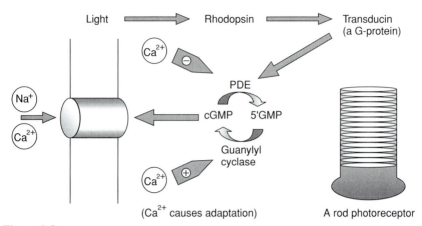

Light ⟹ Rhodopsin ⟹ Transducin (a G-protein)

Ca^{2+} ⊖

PDE

Na^+

cGMP 5'GMP

Ca^{2+}

Guanylyl cyclase

Ca^{2+} ⊕

(Ca^{2+} causes adaptation)

A rod photoreceptor

Figure 6–2

Phototransduction. A rod is depicted at the right, showing the outer segment stacked with disks containing rhodopsin. Light activates rhodopsin, which activates transducin, a specific G-protein. This activates an enzyme (phosphodiesterase, PDE) that breaks down cGMP. Without cGMP inside the rod, the channels close and the rod hyperpolarizes. When the channel closes, less calcium accumulates in the cell. A low level of calcium stimulates guanylyl cyclase and inhibits PDE, leading to increased cGMP.

membrane channels. Thus, photoreceptors are depolarized in the dark, and light causes catalysis of cGMP and a hyperpolarization. Rhodopsin is a G-protein-linked receptor, and, as might be expected, it is a seven transmembrane protein that is homologous with ligand-gated G-protein receptors.

Adaptation The light-stimulated events are reversed in darkness; phosphodiesterase activity declines and guanylate cyclase resumes the formation of cGMP. Light adaptation produces a response that is similar to darkness.

> *Adaptation* results from an abnormally low level of internal calcium that is a direct result of light stimulation.

This low level of calcium increases the activity of guanylate cyclase, suppresses phosphodiesterase activity, and results in a depolarization of the photoreceptor (Figure 6–2). Thus, the photoreceptor's transduction machinery is reset to dark levels despite the presence of background light.

> Calcium plays a key role in photoreceptor adaptation, and it appears to play similar roles in the auditory and olfactory systems.

Rods and Cones

Human photoreceptors can be classified as either *rods* or *cones,* termed a duplex retina. Rods are able to respond to a single photon, whereas cones respond only to hundreds of photons.

Rods also respond more slowly, which means that they can sum the responses to several captured photons. Thus rods are well designed to detect very low levels of light, but they sacrifice both speed and acuity.

Cones are faster; they also are packed more closely together, which means that they have higher spatial resolution (acuity). The fovea, a small central, rod-free region of the retina, has the highest density of cones and therefore the highest acuity. Cones are responsible for color vision, which depends on comparing the relative response of red, green, and blue cones. The response from one color-sensitive cone is subtracted from the other sets of cones in a process termed *color opponency.*

The Neural Retina

The *retina* is a thin slice of tissue that lies inside the back of the eye.

In front of the retina is a gel called the vitreous humor, and in front of this is the lens, then the pupil, the aqueous humor, and the cornea. All of these structures are transparent. Looking into an eye, it is possible to see past all these structures to the black pigment epithelium that is between the neural retina and the sclera (an extension of the cornea that forms the back of the eye).

The retina consists of five major cell types: photoreceptors, horizontal cells, bipolar cells, amacrine cells, and ganglion cells.

The *photoreceptors* are at the back of the retina, so that light must pass through the rest of the neural retina before reaching them. Photoreceptors synapse on *horizontal cells* and two types of *bipolar cells,* ON and OFF. The bipolar cells relay information about the onset and offset of light, respectively, whereas the horizontal cells mediate lateral inhibition between photoreceptors and bipolar cells. Bipolar cells send their signals to the remaining two types of cells: *amacrine cells* and *ganglion cells.* Ganglion cells are responsible for sending information from the retina to various brain regions. Amacrine cells usually suppress, but sometimes enhance, the synaptic signals between bipolar and ganglion cells.

Because of this circuitry, some ganglion cells respond only to light onset and others respond only to light offset. The inhibitory horizontal and amacrine cells produce a center-surround antagonism in ganglion cells. For example, an ON ganglion cell will be depolarized by a light centered over it (covering its dendritic field) but will be inhibited by a light that is peripheral to it (outside its dendritic field). Center-surround antagonism is important for determination of contrast and edge detection. Another type of ganglion cell is directionally selective, responding when a stimulus moves in a particular direction.

Central Pathways

> Signals from the retina go primarily to the *lateral geniculate nucleus* (LGN) in the thalamus and then are relayed to the visual cortex.

In the LGN signals are separated, much as they are in the retina, into a group that detects motion (magnocellular layer) and into another group responsible for color and acuity (parvocellular). The signals from the LGN first reach the primary visual cortex, V1, and then distribute to a number of more specialized processing centers in the visual cortex. The responses in V1 are divided into ocular dominance columns (alternating left and right eye), with an orderly array of orientation-selective cells in each column. The neurons in V1 can be distinguished as (1) *simple,* like the ON and OFF ganglion cells of the retina, (2) *complex,* a mix of ON and OFF responses scattered across the receptive field like a collection of simple cells, and (3) *hypercomplex,* cells that do not respond if light extends beyond the end of their receptive field.

Signals leaving the retina also go to the pretectum, from which they project back to the ciliary body that controls the size of the pupil; to the hypothalamus, to control circadian rhythms; and to the colliculus, to control eye and head movements (saccades and nystagmus, respectively).

Olfaction

Evolutionarily, olfaction is the oldest of the senses.

> Transduction in the *olfactory system* begins when an odorant combines with a receptor, resulting in activation of a G-protein. The receptor cells lie in a sheet of olfactory epithelium that lines the nose.

Olfactory receptor cells are degraded and replaced, an unusual property in sensory receptors but a requirement because of their exposure to the external environment. Unlike the visual system, in which the light spectrum is decomposed into three primary colors, there are about 2000 different odorant receptors, each specialized for the detection of a particular chemical. One hypothesis is that there is a labeled line, whereby each odorant receptor neuron connects to a particular location in the olfactory bulb, and this dedicated circuit identifies the odor.

Olfactory Transduction

> The *olfactory epithelium* consists of a tissue layer made of several cell types: receptor neurons, mucosal cells, and supporting cells.

The receptor neurons are bipolar cells: one end contains odorant receptor proteins in the olfactory cilia that reach into the mucous layer and the other end has an unmyelinated axon sending signals to the brain (Figure 6–3). The ends of olfactory cilia contain specialized receptor proteins (seven transmembrane receptors) that recognize odorants. Each receptor neuron recognizes a specific odorant or a select few odorants. The sensitivity to an odorant depends on its lipid solubility and vapor pressure, ranging from nanomolar to millimolar thresholds of

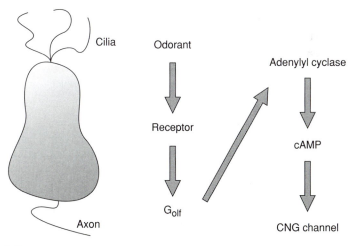

Figure 6–3
An olfactory receptor cell is shown at the left. Receptor proteins are contained in the cilia. Odorants activate these receptors, resulting in activating a G-protein-mediated increase in cAMP. This cyclic nucleotide opens cyclic nucleotide-gated (CNG) channels and depolarizes the cell.

detection. Receptor stimulation leads to G-protein activation. There are two different G-protein transduction pathways in the olfactory system. Most commonly, an odorant binds to a receptor, resulting in stimulation of a G-protein called G_{olf}. This leads to activation of adenylate cyclase and production of cAMP (Figure 6–3), which activates a cyclic nucleotide-gated channel (similar to the channel in photoreceptor cells) that is permeable to monovalent and divalent cations. However, odorant interaction with other receptors may stimulate a different G-protein, leading to activation of phospholipase C, forming inositol triphosphate (IP_3) and elevating the level of internal calcium. Some odorants act primarily through cAMP and others may act through IP_3.

Olfactory Receptors The dynamic range of the olfactory sensory cell is usually less than two orders of magnitude. This would tend to produce a near-binary response from the receptor cell, which does not correlate with behaviorial studies that indicate animals can detect a large range of odorant concentrations. The explanation may be that other odorant receptors not specialized to detect the particular odor nevertheless become active when high concentrations of the odor are encountered.

> Low levels of an odorant are detected by specific receptors, whereas high levels of an odorant are detected by other receptors that are ideally designed to detect a different, but related odor.

Adaptation Adaptation occurs in the olfactory receptor and is probably the result of elevated levels of internal calcium that suppress the formation of cAMP and reduce the affinity of the cyclic nucleotide-gated channel for cAMP. Recovery from adaptation requires several minutes.

Central Pathways

> Signals from olfactory receptors go directly to the olfactory bulb, located in the forebrain.

The axons of olfactory receptor neurons pass through the cribriform plate behind the nose and then synapse on mitral cells in the olfactory bulb. Within the olfactory bulb there are two rows of glomeruli, which are spherical arrays of neuropil that serve as the unit of olfactory information. There is probably one bilateral pair of glomeruli for each odorant. In each glomerulus, tens of mitral cells receive input from thousands of olfactory receptor axons, and mitral cell axons send signals to the rest of the brain. The axons of the mitral cells form the lateral olfactory tract, the primary target of which is the pyriform cortex. The glomerulus also contains several types of interneurons: tufted cells, periglomerular cells, and granule cells.

Taste

The gustatory system contains receptors for a variety of chemicals, which have been difficult to categorize.

One useful classification of the *gustatory system* involves a division of five tastes: sour, salty, bitter, sweet, and umami. These five tastes have clear utility.

Salt detection is important for electrolyte balance, sweet detection is important for energy consumption, sour and bitter detection is an indicator of food quality, and umami detection may provide nutritional information.

Taste receptors are localized to microvilli at the apical tips of taste cells, which are clustered in taste buds throughout the oral cavity, particularly the tongue.

There are about 50–150 taste receptor cells clustered in a taste bud. Because these receptor cells are exposed to the environment, they have a life span of a few weeks. These taste receptor cells are innervated by several cranial nerves that project to the gustatory nucleus in the solitary tract of the medulla. Stimulation of taste receptor cells leads to a synaptic depolarization of the cranial sensory nerves.

Gustatory Transduction

The process of transduction differs for each taste (Figure 6–4). The simplest process seems to be the detection of table salt, NaCl. Salt receptor cells contain constitutively open sodium channels. Consequently, whenever the concentration of salt increases in the oral cavity, sodium ions rush into and depolarize the taste receptor cells. This transduction system is not very sensitive and therefore detects only millimolar changes in salt concentration. These constitutively open channels are blocked by amiloride, and behavioral studies indicate that amiloride interferes with salt taste perception.

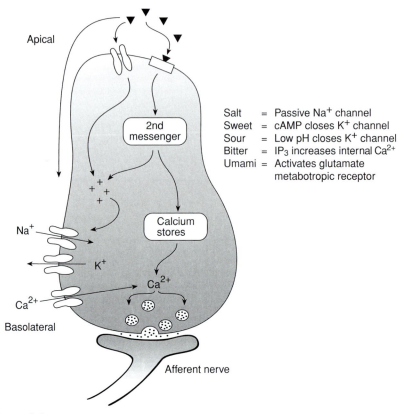

Salt = Passive Na^+ channel
Sweet = cAMP closes K^+ channel
Sour = Low pH closes K^+ channel
Bitter = IP_3 increases internal Ca^{2+}
Umami = Activates glutamate metabotropic receptor

Figure 6–4
Taste receptor cells are found in taste buds in the oral cavity. Stimulation of the receptor proteins leads to release of transmitter, which excites the innervating neurons. Receptor proteins for different tastes use a variety of transduction mechanisms.

The detection of sour tastes depends on the pH sensitivity of potassium channels in sour receptor cells. These potassium channels close in the presence of acidic tastants, resulting in a depolarization of the receptor cell.

The detection of sweet tastes such as sucrose occurs through the tastant's activation of a G-protein receptor, resulting in formation of cAMP. The cAMP closes a potassium channel, thereby depolarizing the taste receptor cell.

Bitter taste is transduced by a G-protein-coupled receptor that activates phospholipase C and production of IP_3. This stimulates the receptor cell by increasing internal calcium, which initiates transmitter release.

Umami taste receptors detect glutamate. Evidence suggests that a particular metabotropic (seven transmembrane) glutamate receptor (termed mGluR4) may encode the umami taste.

The transduction mechanisms in taste receptors are far from resolved, and the outline provided above represents a work in progress. Several G-protein-associated receptors have been identified, but their role in taste transduction is unclear. Gustducin is a G-protein-linked receptor that is analogous to transducin and has been associated with bitter taste receptors. Mice with gustducin knockouts have impaired detection of bitter tastes, but also of sweet tastes. Two other seven transmembrane receptors have been identified: TR1 and TR2. TR1 has been localized to sweet taste buds and TR2 has been localized to bitter taste buds. But neither TR1 nor TR2 is found in taste receptor cells that express gustducin.

In fact, taste reception is more complex than the five-receptor system described. For example, there are amino acid receptors: some activate ligand-gated receptors and others activate G-protein-linked receptors (such as umami receptors). Also, a single taste may have multiple transduction mechanisms. A cAMP pathway transduces the sweet taste of sugar, but the sweet sensation produced by saccharin relies on an IP_3 transduction mechanism.

Auditory System

> The *auditory system* encodes sound, which is a pressure wave that varies in amplitude (loudness) and frequency (pitch).

To detect the high-frequency end of the audible spectrum, which is about 20 kHz in humans and 100 kHz in bats, receptors must distinguish events that occur once every 10–50 millionths of a second. This precludes a chemical transduction mechanism such as the G-protein system. Instead, the system must involve direct, mechanical linkage.

Auditory Transduction

> *Auditory receptors* line the cochlea of the inner ear in humans where they are aligned tonographically according to their sensitivity to frequency.

Receptors sensitive to high-frequency sound waves are proximal and receptors sensitive to low-frequency sound waves are distal. The specialization that allows these receptors to detect sound waves involves a collection of *ciliated cells,* called *hair cells.* The modified cilia, called *stereocilia,* on the apical surface of each hair cell are ordered according to cilium length. In addition, the distal ends of neighboring cilia are connected by a thin fiber called a *tip link.* The tip link fiber appears to be directly connected to a stretch-activated, mechanically gated channel at the tip of the cilium. The bending of stereocilia by sound waves alters the tension that the tip link applies to the gating mechanism of channels at the tips of the cilia (Figure 6–5). The sterocilia are aligned so that movement in one direction increases tension and increases the probability of mechanoreceptor channel openings, whereas pressure in the other direction reduces tension and channels close. Bending this bundle of cilia in the direction of the tallest cilium increases tension and bending in the opposite direction reduces tension on the tip link.

> Thus, bending the cilia increases tension, which opens the channels, or removes tension, which closes the channels.

These pressure-sensitive channels are mechanoreceptors, and their activation leads to a depolarization of the hair cell. When the hair bundle is at rest, a small

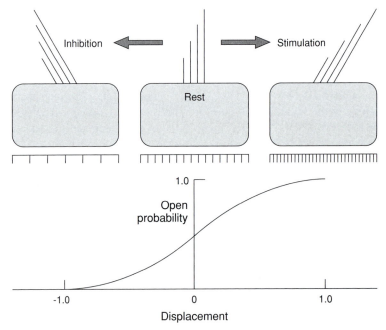

Figure 6–5
Auditory cells contain cilia at their apical surface. Pressure that deflects the cilia in one direction increases tip link tension, activates mechanoreceptor channels, depolarizes the hair cell, and increases spiking; movement in the other direction has the opposite effects.

but significant number of mechanoreceptor channels are open so that the hair cell is slightly depolarized. The activity in the resting state allows the hair cell to alter its spike activity with displacement in either direction, although displacement in the depolarizing direction produces a larger response.

Adaptation Like photoreceptors,

hair cells exhibit adaptation that is dependent on levels of internal calcium.

In this case, stimulation of the stereocilia leads to an influx of calcium through the mechanoreceptors at the distal tip of the stereocilium, and this initiates movement of the tip link–anchoring assembly down the cilium. An actin–myosin interaction may permit this travel of the anchoring mechanism. The result is a loss of tension on the stretch receptor and closing of the mechanoreceptor channel.

Tonotopic Organization

The hair cells are tonotopically arranged along the basilar membrane.

Many properties of hair cells vary depending on the position of the hair cell along the length of the basilar membrane, so that hair cells near the apex are ideally suited to respond to low frequencies and hair cells at the basal end respond to high frequencies. Stereocilium length in the hair cells varies tonotopically, so that long stereocilia are found in hair cells that respond best to low frequencies. Hair cells in lower vertebrates have channels with kinetics that vary according to their position along the basilar membrane. Fast-responding channels are associated with high-frequency-sensitive hair cells. In mammals, the physical characteristics of the basilar membrane result in low-frequency stimuli maximally flexing the membrane near the apex, which is the region most sensitive to low-frequency sound, and higher-frequency stimuli maximally displacing the membrane near the basal section. The tuning by the basilar membrane is facilitated by outer hair cells, which act as piezoelectric devices to change their length during basilar membrane displacement.

In combination, these stimuli activate the inner hair cells, which send auditory information to the brain through the eighth cranial nerve.

Somatosensory System

A variety of stimuli are detected by specialized receptors located on the skin, termed *somatosensory receptors*. Somatosensory receptors, which have their cell bodies in the dorsal root of the spinal cord, send signals through various ascending tracts in the spinal cord to the brainstem and thalamus, and finally to the somatosensory cortex located in the parietal lobe.

The simplest of these somatosensory receptors is free nerve endings that serve as nociceptors and thermoceptors. In addition, there are several specialized, encapsulated mechanoreceptors such as Merkel disks and Ruffini, Meissner, and Pacinian corpuscles. These encapsulated receptors have low thresholds and fast myelinated fibers, permitting a rapid response. Meissner corpuscles and Pacinian corpuscles are rapidly adapting receptors that detect dynamic (transient) changes. The former is designed to detect low-frequency-changes associated with texture, and the latter is designed to detect higher-frequency vibrations and fine texture. There are also slowly adapting (sustained) Merkel disks that detect slow pressure changes associated with detection of shapes, edges, etc. The function of Ruffini corpuscles has not been established. Encapsulated mechanoreceptors are not restricted to the skin. Ruffini corpuscles can be found in ligaments and tendons, and Pacinian corpuscles can be found in the gut. Therefore, these receptors may also serve as proprioceptors, in combination with muscle spindles and Golgi tendon organs, discussed in previous chapters.

Nociceptors

Nociceptors (pain receptors), surprisingly, conduct signals more slowly than encapsulated fibers because they consist of either slightly myelinated ($A\delta$) or unmyelinated (C fibers) axons.

Nociceptors fall into three groups: (1) those that respond only to mechanical stimuli, (2) those that respond to mechanical or thermal stimuli, and (3) polymodal receptors that respond to mechanical, thermal, or chemical stimuli. The first two groups form the $A\delta$ fibers; the polymodal receptors are the slowest, the C fibers.

Nociceptors have a high threshold, responding to the intensity of painful stimuli.

At this level of stimulation, the encapsulated receptors have already been saturated. Thus, an intense stimulus could be carried by both encapsulated and free nerve endings, but the encapsulated endings would convey information about the strength of the stimulus, whereas the free nerve endings would relay information indicating that the stimulus was painful. Among the nociceptors, the Aδ fibers have a lower threshold and convey sharp pain, whereas the C fibers have a higher threshold and convey a duller but more prolonged pain signal.

· C H A P T E R · 7 ·

NEURAL CONTROL OF MOTOR ACTIVITIES

·

Beverly P. Bishop

Motor Innervation of Skeletal Muscles

CNS Control of Muscles

· · · · · · · · · · · ·

MOTOR INNERVATION OF SKELETAL MUSCLES

Movement is a property that distinguishes animals from plants.

In multicellular animals, the *motor system,* which controls movement, involves complex cellular interactions between the skeletal muscles in the periphery and the spinal or brain stem motoneurons, which innervate them.

Activation or suppression of this complex neuromuscular machinery is controlled by excitatory or inhibitory mechanisms operating over the length of the neural axis.

134

Development of Effectors

Myogenesis During embryogenesis, skeletal muscle cells differentiate from mesoderm independently of neurons that differentiate from neuroectoderm.

> During *myogenesis,* the differentiation and development of skeletal muscle proceed in three stages prior to innervation (Figure 7–1A). In the first stage the cell is called a *myoblast,* in the second a *myotube,* and in the third a *myofiber.*

Each stage involves changes in the structure, biochemistry, and excitability of the differentiating cells. Progenitors of all skeletal muscle cells, called presumptive myoblasts, are mononucleated cells capable of synthesizing DNA and dividing mitotically. Myoblasts are capable of fusing with other myoblasts or with myotubes before undergoing further differentiation to become ultimately myofibers (i.e., skeletal muscle cells). Myotube formation requires that myoblasts align with and adhere to each other before fusion (Figure 7–1B). The fusion of myoblasts,

A. Stages in myogenesis

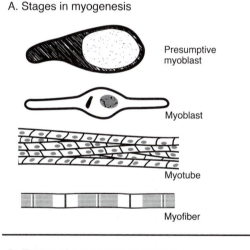

B. Fusion of myoblast and myotube

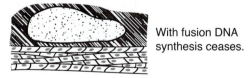

Figure 7–1
(**A**) Stages in maturation of skeletal muscle cells. (**B**) To fuse, a myoblast aligns itself with a myotube.

which involves cadherins, integrins, and neural cell adhesion molecules (NCAMs), creates long, multinucleated cells called myotubes. Most nuclei of myotubes are arranged in single file.

> Fusion triggers many enzymatic and structural changes within the cell.

The enzymes for synthesizing DNA are lost, the synthesis of DNA stops, and, hence, cell division ceases. The cell starts synthesizing contractile filaments (Figure 7–2A). The thin filaments of actin are formed in the cell's periphery, and the thick filaments of myosin form centrally. As myotubes undergo further maturation, the filaments move to positions that form the orderly, precise latticework array that is one characteristic of the structure of skeletal muscle (Figure 7–2B). Z-lines, T-tubules, terminal cisternae, and the sarcoplasmic reticular system gradually appear as the myofiber undergoes further differentiation. Throughout these maturational changes the mitochondria are undergoing changes in their ultrastructure and enzymatic composition. Concurrently Na^+ and K^+ voltage-gated ionic channels and chemically gated acetylcholine receptors (AChRs) appear in

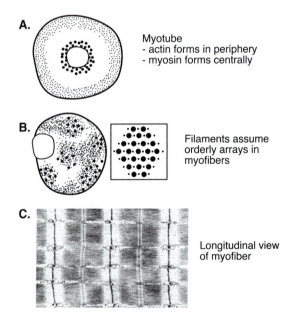

A. Myotube
- actin forms in periphery
- myosin forms centrally

B. Filaments assume orderly arrays in myofibers

C. Longitudinal view of myofiber

Figure 7–2
(**A**) Cross-section of a myotube starting to synthesize the thin contractile filaments of actin centrally and the thick filaments of myosin peripherally. (**B**) With maturation the contractile filaments gradually move together (left) to form precise orderly arrays (right). (**C**) A longitudinal view of a myofiber showing Z-lines, sarcomeres, and striations (characteristic of skeletal muscle).

the cell membrane. Consequently, the cell progressively acquires a resting membrane potential and chemical excitability to acetylcholine.

Spinal Cord Development

Neurogenesis

During *neurogenesis* the position of a cell along the anterior/posterior and dorsal/ventral axes of the neural plate is a determinant of the eventual fate of the cell by virtue of early and positionally restricted inductive signals to which it is exposed.

At the spinal cord and brain stem levels distinct cell types appear at different dorsal/ventral positions. With the formation of the *neural plate,* signaling events initiate the patterning of the spinal cord and the brain stem from the posterior regions of the neural plate (Figure 7–3A).

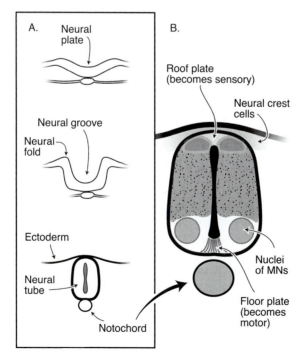

Figure 7–3
(**A**) Ontogeny of the neural tube. (**B**) Regionalization of the neural tube. MNs, motoneurons.

> Morphological changes occur as the result of differential rates of cell growth in the neural plate causing the formation of the *neural folds* and the *neural groove*. Fusion of the neural folds gives rise early in development to the *neural tube*.

Regionalization Within the Primitive Neural Tube

> With fusion of the neural folds, the dorsal region of the newly formed *neural tube* comes into contact with the overlying ectoderm, which appears to be the source of a dorsalizing signal that induces the formation of the *roof plate* and *neural crest*.

Cells migrate from this dorsal region of the neural tube to form the neural crest. These cells ultimately form dorsal root ganglia and several other types of peripheral neural ganglia. Cells within the roof plate region assume sensory function due to the expression of members of the bone morphogenetic protein (BMP) family.

Cells at the midline of the primitive neural plate are in close contact with the mesodermal cells of the notochord (Figure 7–3B). After fusion of the neural folds, the region near the notochord becomes the ventral half of the neural tube. In mutant mice lacking a notochord or in embryos in which the notochord has been surgically removed, neither a floor plate nor motoneurons form.

> The notochord is essential for *floor-plate formation* and *motoneuron differentiation* through the expression of Sonic Hedgehog (SHH).

Experimental evidence has revealed that the specification of the floor plate and several distinct classes of motoneurons and interneurons is due to the concentration gradient of SHH. In fact, SHH is the mediator of notochord and floor-plate-derived mediators of the ventralizing inductive signals in vertebrates.

Formation of Motor Nuclei and Motor Columns

> The first indicator of *motoneuron differentiation* is the expression of Isl-1, a member of a family of homeodomain-containing transcription factors.

Isl-1 is expressed only after prospective motoneurons have undergone their final mitotic division. Initially all motoneurons express Isl-1. If Isl-1 expression is eliminated, motoneurons are not generated despite the presence of floor-plate cells. In the absence of Isl-1 expression, prospective motoneurons undergo apoptosis. Mutant mice lacking Isl-1 or chick neural tube explants treated with antisense Isl-1 oligonucleotides do not generate motoneurons even in the presence of a notochord and floor plate.

> Motoneurons destined for similar function aggregate into distinct clusters forming the *motor nuclei* and *cell columns.*

This clustering of the motoneurons, which leads to the acquisition of *motor pool specificity,* is controlled by neurally derived positional signals that are fixed prior to the generation of motoneurons (Figure 7–4). These signals also provide

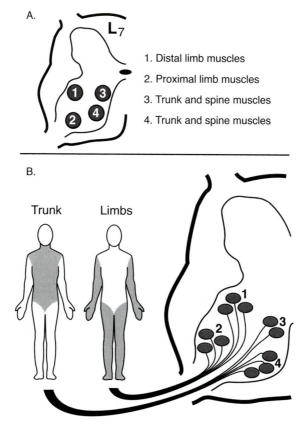

1. Distal limb muscles
2. Proximal limb muscles
3. Trunk and spine muscles
4. Trunk and spine muscles

Figure 7–4
(**A**) Functionally similar cells, ultimately, aggregate into the same nuclei and cell columns. (**B**) Motor pool specificity.

the cues by which an elongating motor axon extends from its discrete motor pool along a muscle-specific pathway to specific muscle cells, its target, in the limb.

Specificity of Innervation

Axonal Elongation, Synaptogenesis, and Cell-to-Cell Interactions (Neurotrophism)   All the neuroblasts within a given motor nucleus will innervate the same muscle. This specificity of innervation occurs prior to axonal elongation or synaptic formation. The spherical neuroblast, on arriving at its appropriate nucleus within the ventral horn, sends out an axon process that grows toward the muscle cells that it will ultimately innervate. (See Chapter 2 for further discussion of the cues used during actual pathfinding.) The growing axon forms a dense arbor near its termination.

> A growth cone on each of these terminal arbors contacts a myofiber, where *synaptogenesis* proceeds (Figure 7–5A). (The events of synaptogenesis are well known. See Chapter 1). The neuroblast in the ventral horn is informed via a retrograde transport about the arrival of growth cones at a target cell (Figure 7–5B). The retrograde signal triggers multiple events that convert the organelles of axon terminals (i.e., the former growth cones) into structures appropriate for a presynaptic ending (Figure 7–5C). The neuron switches from synthesizing materials for axon elongation to synthesizing synaptic vesicles and transmitter (Figure 7–5D).

Maturation of the Neuromuscular Junction and Formation of Motor Units
Although initially more than one synapse may form on a single muscle cell, after a very short postnatal period all *polyneuronal innervation* is lost (Figure 7–6).

> Each muscle cell in a mature muscle receives innervation from one and only one neuron and has just one neuromuscular junction (NMJ). One motoneuron, however, innervates many muscle cells.

A parent axon and all the muscle cells it innervates comprise a *motor unit.* A motor unit operates as an efficient biological amplifier whose output is completely controlled by the firing of its motoneuron.

Concurrently this region of the muscle membrane is undergoing a marked enfolding, meaning that the aggregating AChRs have a larger surface area in which to park. Hence, the muscle membrane under the nerve terminal, the *end plate,* becomes chemically excitable, whereas the extrajunctional part of the mus-

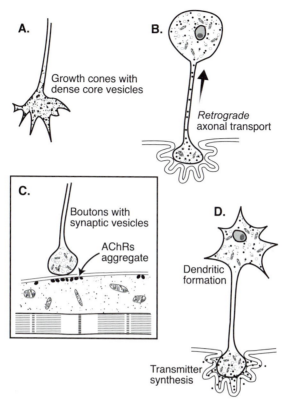

Figure 7–5
(**A**) Elongating axon with growth cones. (**B**) The target signals the axon's arrival by a signal transported retrogradely. (**C**) Growth cones become converted to synaptic boutons. AChRs, acetylcholine receptors. (**D**) Dendrites and synaptic vesicles make their appearance.

cle membrane, from which all AChRs are progressively lost, although retaining its electrical excitability, becomes chemically unexcitable. Concurrently muscle cells are induced to synthesize acetylcholinesterase (AChE), the enzyme that inactivates acetylcholine (ACh) by splitting it into acetate and choline.

Properties of the Neuromuscular Junction

The NMJ, the junction between the motor axon and the muscle cell, is a unique synapse in that sufficient ACh is released to guarantee muscle excitation. Thus, one nerve action potential evokes one muscle action potential.

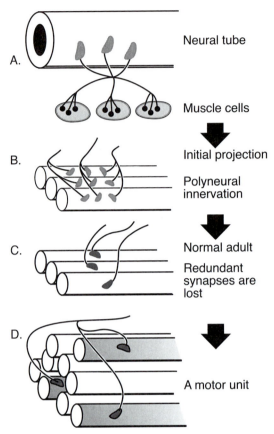

A. Neural tube

Muscle cells

B. Initial projection

Polyneural innervation

C. Normal adult

Redundant synapses are lost

D. A motor unit

Figure 7–6
(**A**) Prior to maturation single muscle fibers may have multiple synapses. (**B**) Polyneuronal innervation persists if muscle activity is eliminated. (**C**) Rate of synapse elimination is enhanced by direct stimulation of motor neurons. (**D**) A motor unit. One axon innervates many muscle cells.

As a consequence the firing frequency of a motor unit accurately reflects that of its motoneuron. Once innervated, a muscle cell becomes a slave to its motoneuron because of the motoneuron's control of the muscle's firing, as just described, and because of the motoneuron's *neurotrophic control* over the well-being of the muscle cell.

The neurotrophic interactions between muscle and motoneuron are a lifelong affair. In the absence of these important cell-to-cell interactions, as would occur following injury or section of a motor axon, both motoneurons and muscles undergo a sequence of dramatic morphological and functional changes.

Motoneuron Responses to Axotomy

Dramatic changes occur in a motoneuron following a lesion to its axon.

These changes include displacement of the nucleus from the center of the soma toward the periphery, a phenomenon histologists call *chromatolysis* (Figure 7–7A), and a loss of central nervous system (CNS) connections (Figure 7–7B). Functionally a surviving neuron switches from synthesizing neural transmitter to

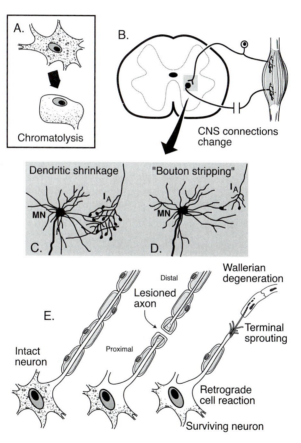

Figure 7–7
(**A**) Following axonal injury a motoneuron's cell nucleus becomes displaced and its cellular organelles assume new functions. (**B**) The motoneuron loses central connections. (**C**) Its dendrites retract. (**D**) Presynaptic terminals of I_A terminals withdraw from the motoneuron. (**E**) A cascade of events occurs in the proximal and distal segments of the lesioned axon during degeneration and reinnervation.

synthesizing axonal membrane. Its dendritic tree undergoes a dramatic shrinkage (Figure 7–7C). Terminal endings of afferent inputs to an injured cell retract, a phenomenon known as *bouton stripping* (Figure 7–7D). The axonal segment distal to the lesion undergoes a phagocytotic sequence of events called *Wallerian degeneration* (Figure 7–7E). If the neuron survives the axonal damage, the axonal segment proximal to the lesion puts out *terminal* or *regenerative sprouts* whose growth cones grow out to reinnervate the denervated target cells (Figure 7–7E). Most aspects of axonal regeneration recapitulate growth cone formation and axonal elongation that occur during ontogeny.

Muscle Responses to the Death of its Motoneuron or to Denervation Due to Axotomy

When the connection between a motoneuron and muscle becomes disrupted due to injury or disease, the muscle becomes flaccid and atrophies.

The contractile and elastic structures within the sarcomeres undergo biochemical, histochemical, and physiological changes. Equally dramatic changes occur in the membrane of a denervated muscle, including mobilization of existing acetylcholine receptors, which move out from the end-plate region, and the insertion of newly synthesized receptors along the entire muscle cell, making the distribution pattern analogous to that of the embryo (Figure 7–8).

CNS CONTROL OF MUSCLES

Recruitment and Rate Coding

Sherrington recognized that the alpha-motoneurons comprise the *final common pathway,* as they exert total control over the muscle fibers they innervate.

CNS control of motor output is mediated in two ways: *recruitment* and *rate coding.*

Recruitment is a course control. During a motor action in which only a weak motor output is required, only a small fraction of the total motor pool is activated or recruited. (The *motor pool* is the total population of neurons innervating a par-

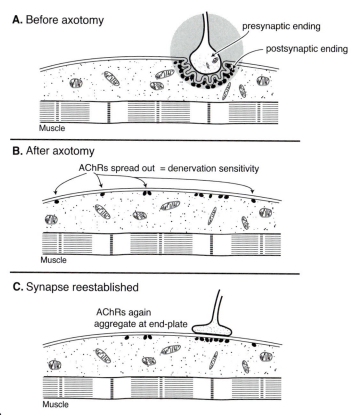

Figure 7–8
(**A**) Synapses before axotomy. (**B**) Changes in receptor distribution after axotomy. AChRs, acetylcholine receptors. (**C**) Reformation of synapse after reinnervation.

ticular muscle.) Neighboring motoneurons within the same motor pool might also be recipients of a small part of the excitatory command, but their depolarization is insufficient to bring the membrane potential to its firing level. Sherrington called this facilitated but unexcited fraction of the motor pool the *subliminal fringe*. With minimal additional excitatory input, these neurons are *recruited* and become part of the *discharge zone*.

Rate coding involves control of the motoneuron's firing frequency and pattern. Many extrinsic and intrinsic factors determine the firing behavior of motoneurons. The final determinants are (1) the level of depolarization [e.g., the amplitude of the excitatory postsynaptic potential (EPSP)], (2) the time course of the depolarization, and (3) the intrinsic characteristics of the ion channels populating the initial segment of the motoneuron.

Motoneuron Types

Alpha-motoneurons fall into two structural and functional categories: *tonic* and *phasic*. *Tonic motoneurons* are small neurons that innervate the slow or red muscles, which perform the sustained contractions that support the body against gravity. *Phasic motoneurons* are large neurons that innervate the fast or pale muscles, which perform quick, short-lasting, ballistic muscle responses.

Small motoneurons are generally recruited earlier than large motoneurons in a reflex response or a voluntary movement. This fact gave rise to the *size principle,* which states that small motor units are recruited before large motor units.

The frequency of discharge for any motoneuron is essentially a linear function of the level of depolarization as shown by the experimental data in Figure 7–9. These data were derived from intracellular recordings made from an alpha-motoneuron while its soma was maintained at a preselected level of depolarization by injected current (an experimental procedure known as voltage clamping). The greater the depolarization (e.g., the larger the EPSP) the higher the firing frequency. The slope of the frequency versus depolarization function depends on the neuron's *gain,* which varies among the various types of motoneurons due to the intrinsic differences in the opening and closing properties of the ionic channels comprising the excitable membrane. (See Chapter 3 for more details.)

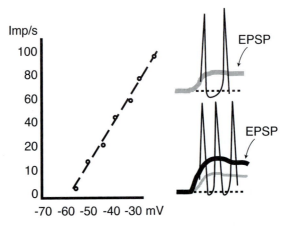

Figure 7–9
The slope of the line (i.e., gain) defining the firing frequency (i.e., the impulses per second) as a function of the level of depolarization varies among neurons. The amplitude and duration of an excitatory postsynaptic potential (EPSP) sets the impulse intervals (i.e., the firing frequency).

Intrinsic Properties Differentiating Tonic and Phasic Alpha-Motoneurons

> At identical levels of depolarization the tonic and phasic alpha-motoneurons differ in the time courses of their after-hyperpolarizations (AHPs) and firing profiles (Figure 7–10).

In response to a sustained depolarization, the AHP of a phasic alpha-motoneuron, because of its shallower trough and steeper depolarizing slope, is shorter than the AHP of a tonic motoneuron. Thus, a phasic motoneuron is capable of a higher firing rate than a tonic motoneuron. The profile of a neuron's AHP is determined by the voltage-dependent sodium and potassium channels populating the cell's excitable membrane.

Hierarchical Levels of Movement Control

How is this peripheral machinery activated to generate coordinated, purposeful movements? It depends on three hierarchical levels of control: (1) the

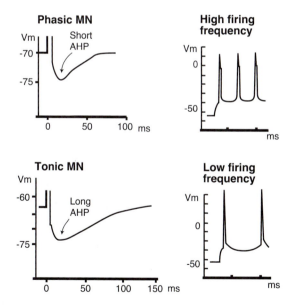

Figure 7–10
An after-hyperpolarization's time course is determined by the intrinsic properties of the ion channels of a motoneuron. The time course, in turn, determines the neuron's firing frequency.

segmental and intersegmental *spinal reflexes,* (2) *brain stem control,* and (3) control by the *cerebral cortex.* Each higher level projects to the spinal cord in parallel.

> Movements fall into three classes: *reflexes, rhythmic motor patterns,* and *voluntary movements.*

Spinal reflexes are discussed in this chapter. Respiration as an example of rhythmic behavior and voluntary motor control are considered in Chapters 8 and 9.

Formation of Spinal Reflex Circuits

Reflexes evolve early in ontogeny.

> Soon after fusion of the neural tube and its subsequent regionalization, the motoneurons establish synaptic connections with muscle cells.

At this time, the fetus generates spontaneous, nonpurposeful movements demonstrating a functional readiness. All types of neurons have made their appearance within the spinal cord, but no central synapses have yet been formed.

> The dorsal root ganglia, formed by neural crest cells, contain neurons destined to become the primary somatosensory cells serving all the cutaneous and proprioceptive senses.

The peripherally directed process of these bipolar cells grows out to innervate appropriate receptors in the skin, muscles, and joints, and the central branch grows into the dorsal horn of the developing neural tube.

Formation of the Flexor Reflex Arc   Among the earliest synapses to form within the spinal cord are those between the central processes of primary sensory neurons, whose afferent fibers comprise groups II, III, and IV, and excitatory interneurons deep in the dorsal horn or in the intermediate lateral gray (Figure 7–11A). These small interneurons, in turn, make excitatory synapses on the alpha-motoneurons controlling the flexor limb muscles.

This disynaptic circuit is the first or most primitive neural arc to be completed in the spinal cord. It is called the *flexor reflex* or the *withdrawal reflex* (Figure 7–11A).

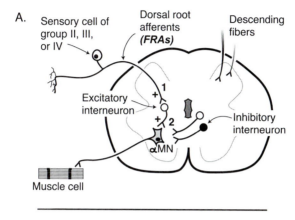

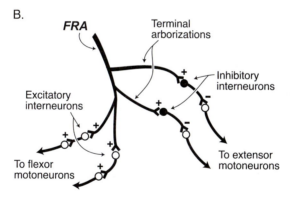

Figure 7–11
(A) Formation of spinal neural connections (1 and 2 indicate *sequence* of synapse formation). The first reflex arc (the flexion reflex) is now complete. αMN, alpha-motoneuron; FRAs, flexor reflex afferents. (B) Reciprocal inhibition: terminal arbors of the FRAs synapse on inhibitory interneurons that suppress extensor motoneuron firing.

Like all primary afferents, the central projections from the dorsal root ganglia send out collateral branches after entering the central gray. In addition to their primary projections to excitatory interneurons, these *flexor reflex afferents* (FRAs) make excitatory synapses on *inhibitory interneurons*. The axons of these inhibitory interneurons project ipsilaterally to the alpha-motoneurons innervating the extensor muscles. This circuitry mediates *reciprocal inhibition,* the function of which is to relax the extensor muscles at the same time the flexor muscles are activated. Hence the limb is permitted to be withdrawn from a noxious stimulus.

Formation of the Crossed Extensor Reflex In addition to this ipsilateral circuitry, the *excitatory interneurons* send collaterals across the midline in the anterior commissure. These contralateral projections form excitatory synapses within the *extensor* alpha motor pool (Figure 7–11B).

> The reflex response mediated by this neural arc is called the *crossed extensor reflex.*

When a stimulated limb is reflexly withdrawn in response to input from the FRAs the contralateral limb is extended. Hence, this crossed extension reflex helps prevent a fall whenever a flexion reflex causes a sudden withdrawal of a stimulated limb.

Formation of the Stretch Reflex Soon after the flexor reflex circuit is established, the central projections of the largest sensory cells in the dorsal root ganglia, the group I_A afferent fibers, unlike any other primary afferent input, grow into and through the central gray to synapse directly on alpha-motoneurons (Figure 7–12). The peripheral branches of these I_A afferents innervate primary endings of the *muscle spindles.* The central projection of each group I_A afferent terminates in a dense arbor and makes excitatory synapses on 90% of the alpha-

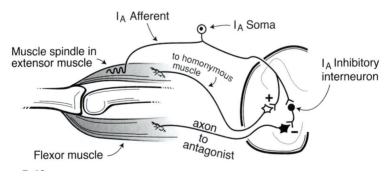

Figure 7–12
I_A afferent fibers make direct contact on alpha-motoneurons to form the monosynaptic reflex arc. Terminal arbors of the same I_A afferent fibers diverge to synapse on inhibitory interneurons; the I_A inhibitory interneurons that, in turn, project to motoneurons innervating the antagonist, another example of reciprocal inhibition.

motoneurons in the motor pool innervating the homonymous (same) muscle in which the spindle resides. Thus, a reflex arc consisting of only one central synapse is formed.

This circuit is known as the *monosynaptic reflex* or the *stretch reflex.* It mediates both the *tonic* and *phasic stretch reflexes.*

The tonic stretch reflexes are essential for maintaining posture; the phasic stretch reflexes provide the neurologist with a useful test for assessing CNS excitability. For example, the neurologist taps the patellar tendon to evoke the *knee jerk reflex.* The tendon tap stretches the quadriceps muscle and the muscle spindles distributed throughout the muscle. This stretch is an adequate stimulus for initiating a brief, high-frequency burst of action potentials in the I_A afferent fibers. In response to this excitatory input, the motoneurons of the quadriceps are briefly activated, and the leg extends.

Muscle Spindles

Muscle spindles are complex sensory structures that are exquisitely responsive to the muscle's absolute (or static) length, change in length, and rate of change in length.

Because these receptors are attached to and lie in parallel with the extrafusal muscle fibers, their length is changed in concert with the length of the muscle. The I_A afferent input increases its firing frequency with an increase in muscle length and slows or ceases firing with a decrease in muscle length. All spindle input is excitatory, and any *passive stretch* of a muscle during movements is signaled by the primary endings of muscle spindles. The alpha motor pool of the stretched muscle is the recipient of this spindle-generated excitation.

Such *autogenous excitation* serves as a negative feedback circuit whose function is to stabilize muscle length.

Any increase in the length of a muscle, as might occur during movement of a joint, causes, via the monosynaptic stretch reflex arc, activation of the stretched muscle, which counteracts the passive stretch.

Reciprocal Inhibition via I_A Interneurons   The central projections of the I_A afferents from the primary spindle endings also project to a population of inhibitory interneurons called I_A *interneurons,* which, in turn, make inhibitory synapses on the alpha-motoneurons innervating muscles antagonistic to the stretched muscle (Figure 7–12). (An antagonistic muscle is a muscle whose action on a joint is opposite to that of an agonist.)

> This neural circuit via the I_A inhibitory interneuron is another example of *reciprocal inhibition.*

Stretching an extensor muscle simultaneously invokes activation of the extensor muscle and suppression of activity in the flexor motoneurons permitting the limb to extend.

Autogenous Inhibition Imposed by Golgi Tendon Organs

> The *Golgi tendon organs* are a group of muscle receptors that signal changes in a muscle's active tension or effort (Figure 7–13).

The primary afferent fibers serving Golgi tendon organs are large group I_B fibers. Early in ontogeny the central projections of these I_B fibers synapse on a population of inhibitory interneurons known as the I_B *inhibitory interneurons,* which, in turn, synapse on the alpha-motoneurons innervating the homonymous

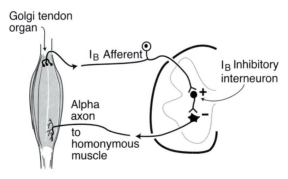

Figure 7–13
The neural circuit imposing *autogenous inhibition,* a polysynaptic reflex initiated by Golgi tendon organ input and operating via I_B inhibitory interneurons.

muscle. Hence, this reflex exerts *autogenous inhibition,* which provides negative feedback that stabilizes tension. Any tension developed by a muscle is counteracted by the I_B-mediated inhibition. Such a reflex circuit limits the voluntary tension that can be achieved and prevents the muscle from developing unsafe tensions.

Recurrent Inhibition Imposed by Renshaw Cells The axons of the alpha-motoneurons put out collateral branches prior to leaving the ventral horn. These axon collaterals make synaptic connections on yet another population of inhibitory interneurons called Renshaw cells (Figure 7–14A).

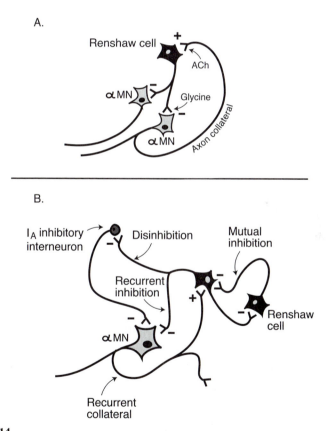

Figure 7–14
(**A**) *Recurrent inhibition.* One Renshaw cell inhibits many alpha-motoneurons (α-MNs) within the same motor pool. ACh, acetylcholine. (**B**) In addition to *recurrent inhibition,* Renshaw cells exert *disinhibition* of alpha-motoneurons by inhibiting I_A inhibitory interneurons and *mutual inhibition* by inhibiting other Renshaw cells.

> *Renshaw cells,* named after the American neurophysiologist who first iden-
> tified them and described their properties, are small, spontaneously active,
> glycinergic interneurons whose major input is from the axon collaterals of
> neighboring alpha-motoneurons.

Renshaw cells increase their firing frequencies in response to alpha-motoneuron input. Because Renshaw cells project to several types of neurons, they have diverse functions. A major Renshaw projection is directed back to the alpha-motoneurons from which it received excitation.

> The faster a motoneuron fires the faster the Renshaw cells fire, and the
> greater the inhibition they exert. Such a neural circuit is an example of
> *recurrent inhibition.*

A single Renshaw cell makes projections to many motoneurons in the same motor pool. The negative feedback imposed by Renshaw cells modifies the firing rate of many alpha-motoneurons. As a consequence of recurrent inhibition, weakly firing motoneurons are silenced; however, the effect exerted on strongly firing motoneurons is not as great. As a result the focus of the discharge zone is sharpened.

Other Projections of Renshaw Cells   Renshaw cells project not only to alpha-motoneurons but to other Renshaw cells and to I_A inhibitory interneurons (Figure 7–14B).

> The result of one inhibitory cell imposing inhibition on another inhibitory
> interneuron is called *disinhibition* (i.e., a target cell normally a recipient of
> inhibition is relieved of that inhibition).

Renshaw cells project to the I_A inhibitory interneurons (i.e., that population of interneurons mediating the reciprocal innervation that accompanies the stretch reflex). Renshaw cells also project to other Renshaw cells to mediate *mutual inhibition.*

Spinal Reflexes Are Hard-Wired and Stable   Once formed, spinal reflex circuits remain remarkably stable throughout life. Compared with neural circuits formed in the brain, spinal reflexes are considerably less labile. Under very carefully controlled experimental conditions, it has been shown that some remodeling (i.e., learning) of the reflex circuits can occur.

> Inhibition is the major mechanism by which the *hard-wired spinal reflexes* are controlled during the learning of complex motor acts.

In conclusion, the hard-wired spinal reflexes provide the fundamental circuitry for postural adjustments and movements throughout life, freeing the brain of menial tasks.

RHYTHMIC MOTOR ACTIVITY AND RESPIRATION

·

Beverly P. Bishop

The Respiratory Pump

Neurons Involved in Respiratory Control

Respiratory Reflexes

Ondine's Curse

THE RESPIRATORY PUMP

Breathing has long been recognized as a tightly controlled rhythmic motor act. Details of the mechanisms by which the nervous system generates the appropriate motor activity to match ventilation exactly to the body's metabolic demands are still being elucidated. Nonetheless, it has long been recognized that respiration during quiet breathing occurs quite automatically, much like spinal reflexes. Yet, it is possible to voluntarily hold one's breath, or control the depth and/or the frequency of breathing for considerable periods, but not indefinitely.

These facts demonstrate that respiration is neither 100% reflexive nor 100% voluntary in nature, but is tightly controlled by sensory feedback.

The respiratory pump acts in an executive capacity setting priorities and directing a great raft of effectors to perform in the right sequence, at the right level, and for the proper duration. Otherwise, ventilation will not be maintained at an appropriate range for the varying levels of metabolism and varying environmental conditions.

Control of respiration requires both a *central pattern generator* (CPG) to control the recruitment of muscles and the sequencing of their activity and a *central rhythm generator* (CRG) to control the timing of this activity.

NEURONS INVOLVED IN RESPIRATORY CONTROL

Like any controlled system,

the *respiratory control system* has three major components: the *controller,* the *controlled elements,* and the *sensors* to provide feedback to the controller.

The *controller* is composed of the central respiratory neurons that initiate respiratory rhythm (CRG) and neurons that govern the order and level of recruitment of the brain stem premotoneurons (CPG). The axons of these premotoneurons project to the spinal alpha-motoneurons innervating the pump muscles including the diaphragm and the muscles of the chest and abdominal wall, which produce inspiration and expiration.

The Controlled Elements or Effectors

The major *inspiratory muscle* is the *diaphragm,* which is innervated by the right and left phrenic nerves, each of which projects unilaterally.

Phrenic motoneurons are recruited for each *inspiration* throughout life. Contraction of the diaphragm creates a negative pressure within the lung and chest causing an inward flow of air. The volume of air that moves into the lung depends on the pressure generated by the respiratory muscles, which is partially determined by the level of recruitment and the duration of contraction of the diaphragm. During quiet breathing, *expiration* is accomplished in large part by the elastic recoil of the lungs and chest wall with little need for recruitment of expiratory motoneurons. When breathing becomes augmented, as during exercise, the motoneurons innervating the *expiratory muscles* (i.e., the internal intercostals of the chest wall and the abdominal muscles) are recruited rhythmically out of phase with the diaphragm.

The Central Rhythm Generator

The source of this vital rhythmic motor activity has intrigued investigators for a century. Serial transections of a cat brain stem, performed in a rostral-to-caudal direction, defined the level of the neural axis at which respiratory rhythm is generated. Figure 8–1 shows the results of these experiments. Following a transection at the rostral border of the pons in an anesthetized cat, the normal breathing pattern is not disrupted. Following a mid-pontine transection, however, the breathing pattern becomes *apneustic,* which means that the inspirations are deep and prolonged. Hence, the rostral pons exerts some control over the breathing pattern. However, the pons is *not* responsible for rhythmic respiration as breathing persists following a mid-pontine transection. Following a transection between the pons and medulla, the breathing pattern reverts to a pattern very close to normal, demonstrating that

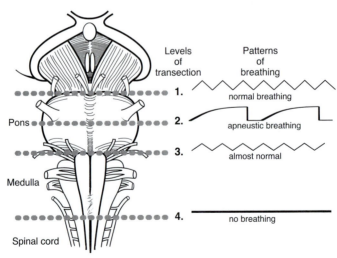

Figure 8–1
Results of brain stem transections at sequential levels (1 through 4) demonstrated that the crucial neurons for rhythmic respiration lie within the medulla between levels 3 and 4. Spinal neurons in the absence of descending input have *no* spontaneous rhythm.

the primary rhythm generator must still be functional. In marked contrast, when the brain stem transection is located between the medulla and the spinal cord, all breathing is abolished. These results reveal two important points.

First, the crucial neurons for the maintenance of rhythmic respiratory activity lie within the medulla somewhere between the pons and spinal cord. Second, the spinal motoneurons innervating the respiratory muscles possess no intrinsic rhythmicity.

Identifying Central Neurons with Respiratory Function

Results of the serial transections of the brain stem raised essential questions about which medullary neurons have respiratory function and where or how the respiratory rhythm is generated. Criteria to determine whether a brain stem neuron is a respiratory neuron are determined from recordings made from single medullary neurons (Figure 8–2).

Any medullary neuron that discharges in phase with phrenic motor activity or the diaphragm EMG is labeled an I-neuron (I for inspiratory). Any neuron whose depolarization is out of phase with phrenic activity and whose hyperpolarization is in phase with the phrenic or diaphragm discharge is considered an E-neuron (E for expiration).

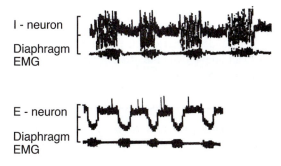

Figure 8–2
Criteria for determining whether a brain stem neuron is a respiratory-related neuron and, if so, determining the respiratory phase to which its discharge is phase locked. Upper traces: an I-neuron discharging in phase with the diaphragm. Lower traces: an E-neuron discharging out of phase with the diaphragm. EMG, electromyogram.

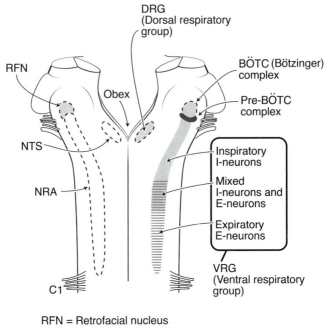

DRG
(Dorsal respiratory group)

RFN

Obex

BÖTC (Bötzinger) complex

Pre-BÖTC complex

NTS

Inspiratory I-neurons

NRA

Mixed I-neurons and E-neurons

Expiratory E-neurons

VRG
(Ventral respiratory group)

C1

RFN = Retrofacial nucleus
NTS = Nucleus tractus solitarius
NRA = Nucleus retroambigualis
C1 = 1st cervical nerve

Figure 8–3
Locations of the central respiratory neurons. Anatomical sites are on the left. Functional types of respiratory-related neurons are on the right. (See text for details.)

Such designations, of course, provide information only about the timing of the neuron's activity and not about the neuron's projections or functions. To answer the first question requires identification of the location of I-neurons and E-neurons. Figure 8–3 shows diagrammatically the gross locations of the major populations of central respiratory neurons.

> These include the *Bötcinger complex,* the *pre-Bötcinger complex,* the *dorsal respiratory group,* and the *ventral respiratory group.*

The Bötcinger Complex   The Bötcinger complex (BÖTC) is a group of inhibitory neurons lying rostral to the nucleus retroambigualis (NRA) and corresponding anatomically to the retrofacial nucleus (RFN) (Figure 8–3).

> BÖTC neurons fire in phase with expiration, making them E-neurons.

They are reputed to exert strong reciprocal inhibition even during quiet breathing. This inhibition is directed to the pontine respiratory group (PRG) and to most other groups of respiratory-related neurons in the brain stem. They do not, however, project to the spinal cord.

The Dorsal Respiratory Group Anatomically the dorsal respiratory group (DRG) lies very close to the nucleus tractus solitarius (NTS), the major site of termination of visceral afferent fibers from cranial nerves IX and X. NTS contains the second-order neurons that ascend from the brain stem to the thalamus.

> DRG neurons are of two types: *I-neurons* and *P-cells,* neither of which has any intrinsic rhythm.

The *I-neurons* of the DRG are premotoneurons that project to contralateral phrenic motoneurons. The *P-cells* (pump cells) are small neurons that derive their name from the fact that they discharge in phase with lung inflation induced by a mechanical ventilator. P-cells are not premotoneurons in that they do not project to the spinal cord, but rather are inhibitory interneurons that project locally within the brain stem. They are involved in respiratory reflexes, which will be discussed subsequently.

The Ventral Respiratory Group The ventral respiratory group (VRG) extends over the entire longitudinal length of the NRA from the rostral to the caudal medulla. In the absence of afferent input, recordings from VRG neurons lack intrinsic rhythm. Thus, the VRG cannot be the source of respiratory rhythm.

> I-neurons are clustered in the *rostral* end of the VRG, and E-neurons are concentrated in the *caudal* end.

E-neurons and I-neurons are intermixed in the *middle* region of the VRG (Figure 8–4). All VRG neurons project to the PRG of neurons and cross near the obex to project to the respiratory-related neurons in the contralateral VRG and the spinal cord.

I-neurons of the rostral VRG are subdivided into *early-burst I-neurons,* whose peak firing frequency occurs early in the inspiratory phase, and *late-peak I-neurons,* whose firing starts late in inspiration (Figure 8–4).

The early-burst I-neurons make no spinal projections, but they do project to the opposite VRG to synapse over the entire length of the contralateral NRA. In contrast, the late-peak I-neurons project to respiratory-related neurons in the contralateral C4 and T12 levels of the spinal cord.

E-neurons of the *caudal VRG* cross at a level caudal to the obex and project to expiratory motoneurons in the spinal cord (Figure 8–4). To date, these VRG E-neurons are the only known premotor respiratory neurons that project to and

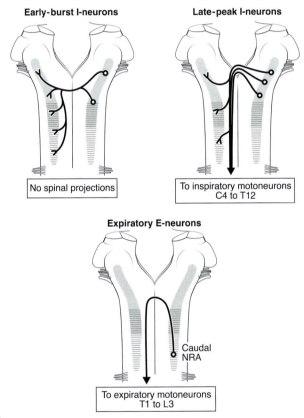

Figure 8–4
VRG neurons are grouped into types based on the timing of their activity in the respiratory cycle and their projections to other brain stem neurons and to the spinal cord.

control the spinal expiratory motoneurons. In other words, these expiratory VRG premotoneurons provide the major, if not the only, descending neural control of the expiratory activity in the spinal abdominal motoneurons. These premotor E-neurons appear to be involved in all the diverse functions of the abdominal muscles including sound production and expulsive maneuvers such as defecation, micturition, parturition, and vomiting.

Where is Respiratory Rhythm Generated?

Because none of the neurons in the Bötcinger complex, the DRG, or the VRG possesses any intrinsic rhythmic activity, the major questions of where and how respiratory rhythm is generated remained unanswered for decades. Recently novel experimental preparations have been introduced that have provided new clues as to the source of respiratory rhythm. Among these useful preparations is the *isolated brain stem–spinal cord* from neonatal rat. Spontaneous rhythmic activity persists in this isolated preparation in a brain stem region just caudal to the BÖTC (Figure 8–3) and rostral to the VRG.

> This region, which is close to the caudal retrotrapezoid nucleus (RTN), is known as the *pre-Bötcinger complex* (pre-BÖTC).

Rostral-to-caudal serial microsections (every ~200 μm) of the RTN have precisely localized the pre-BÖTC. Recordings of spontaneous activity from neurons in this region display a rhythm that correlates with that of the hypoglossal nucleus whose motoneurons, like the phrenic motoneurons, discharge with each inspiration.

Medullary brain slices ~500-μm thick are proving to be another useful preparation for analyzing the intrinsic properties of neurons in the pre-BÖTC. Whole cell, patch clamp, voltage clamp, and synaptic current recordings from these rhythmically active neurons, before and after pharmacological blocking, have been obtained and analyzed. Results from diverse experimental paradigms have revealed that

> the neurons in the pre-BÖTC region possess *voltage-dependent, pacemaker-like properties.*

Depolarization of the pre-BÖTC (by elevating the external K^+ concentration) results in a bilateral elevation of the burst frequency. Blocking glutaminergic synapses in the pre-BÖTC reduces burst frequency and transiently blocks rhythmo-genesis.

> All of the following experimental findings support the hypothesis that the *pre-BÖTC* is the most likely source of respiratory rhythm.

Neurons in this complex have an intrinsically generated rhythm. Ablation of this complex in an otherwise intact animal causes cessation of respiration. Pharmacological blocking of non-N-methyl-D-aspartate receptors in this complex transiently abolishes respiratory rhythm. The rhythm-generating neurons of the pre-BÖTC are interneurons that do not project outside the bulbar region. Rather they project to the bulbospinal premotoneurons. Pre-BÖTC neurons are responsive to hypercapnia and, in fact, are closely associated with many of the chemoreceptor functions attributed to the rostral ventrolateral medulla.

RESPIRATORY REFLEXES

A large variety of sensory inputs project to the central respiratory neurons (Figure 8–5).

> Chemosensors lying in the periphery and in the brain stem near the central respiratory neurons have powerful control over respiration.

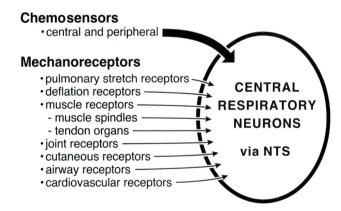

Figure 8–5
Many types of sensory inputs modulate the activity of the central respiratory neurons. NTS, nucleus tractus solitarius.

After all, the major physiological purpose of ventilation is to maintain the homeostasis of O_2 and CO_2 and the pH of arterial blood, cerebral spinal fluid (CSF), and extracellular fluid.

> Any increase in arterial CO_2 increases ventilation and any decrease in arterial CO_2 decreases ventilation. In fact, ventilation has been shown to require chemical stimulation.

When the CO_2 produced by an animal is experimentally removed without disrupting the delivery of O_2, the animal ceases breathing (Figure 8–6). Because the chemostatus of the blood and/or of the CSF exerts such a strong influence over respiration, we need to know where the chemosensors are and how they exert their influence. CO_2 is sensed both centrally and peripherally. Although sites on the ventrolateral surface of the medulla have been identified as chemosensitive, no specific cells have been identified as being endowed with unique chemosensing properties. Nonetheless, it is accepted that changes in the CO_2 and pH in the arterial blood and the central spinal fluid initiate appropriate modulations in the breathing pattern that bring the CO_2 and pH levels toward normal.

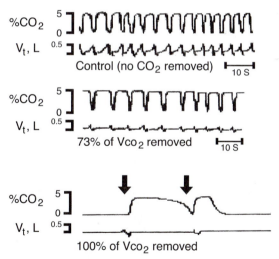

Figure 8–6
Removal of CO_2 from venous blood stopped ventilation! When prodded (at arrows) the sheep was capable of breathing. V_t, tidal volume in liters; $\dot{V}_{CO_2}$, carbon dioxide production. (From E.A. Phillipson et al., *J Appl Physiol* 1981;50:45–54.)

Chemoreflexes

Peripheral chemoreceptors have been characterized in considerable more detail than the central sensors. The peripheral receptors lie in the carotid and aortic bodies close to the heart (Figure 8–7A). These sites position them to "taste" the arterial blood before it reaches the central respiratory neurons.

> Among the cells in the aortic and carotid bodies are unique cells that serve as O_2 sensors.

Whereas a fall in arterial oxygen depresses most neural cells, it excites the peripheral chemoreceptors.

The transduction steps whereby a fall in arterial oxygen is converted to action potentials in cranial nerve IX are shown in Figure 8–7B. The glomus cells of the carotid body contain special potassium channels that are oxygen sensitive.

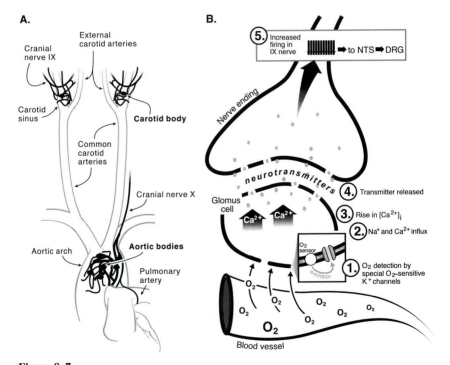

Figure 8–7
(**A**) Location of the peripheral chemoreceptors in the carotid and aortic bodies. (**B**) Transduction steps in the carotid body. NTS, nucleus tractus solitarius; DRG, dorsal respiratory group.

A decrease in O_2 tension opens these channels, permitting an elevation of intracellular K^+. As a consequence the concentration of intracellular calcium rises. (The source or mechanism of this rise in intracellular calcium is still being debated.)

The *glomus cell* in response to the increase in $[Ca^{2+}]_i$ mobilizes and releases neurotransmitter, which binds to receptors on the afferent nerve terminal opening channels that lead to depolarization and action potential generation.

The afferent fibers of cranial nerve IX conduct these impulses to the nucleus tractus solitarius (NTS) and from those onto DRG neurons.

An elevation of CO_2 in the inspired gas mixture or any physiological condition that permits end-title CO_2 to rise to 10% or higher excites both peripheral and central chemoreceptors, causing ventilation to increase.

The hyperpolarization of the glomus cells during expiration and the depolarization during inspiration are greater during hypercapnia than during eucapnia. This hypercapnic enhancement of the magnitude of the fluctuations in carotid body membrane potentials accounts for the augmented firing frequency in the afferent fibers.

Vagal-Mediated Mechanoreflexes

Mechanoreceptors, whose signals provide continuous feedback to central respiratory neurons by way of the vagus nerve, are located along the length of the airway from the extra- and intrathoracic upper airways to the smallest terminal bronchi. Signals from these mechanoreceptors are propagated to the brain stem by afferent fibers in the vagus nerve (i.e., cranial nerve X). The cell bodies of these vagal neurons lie in the nodose ganglia, whose central projections terminate in the medial, intermediate, and ventrolateral subnuclei of the NTS in the vicinity of the DRG. These vagal inputs evoke two types of respiratory reflexes: *regulatory* and *defensive* (or *protective*) reflexes.

The mechanoreceptors giving rise to these two types of reflexes are of two functional types based on their adaptation characteristics: *slowly adapting receptors* (SARs) and *rapidly adapting receptors* (RARs) (Figure 8–8).

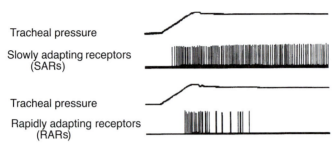

Tracheal pressure

Slowly adapting receptors (SARs)

Tracheal pressure

Rapidly adapting receptors (RARs)

Figure 8–8
Distinguishing characteristics in the discharge patterns of the slowly adapting receptors (SARs) and the rapidly adapting receptors (RARs) recorded from pulmonary mechanoreceptors in response to an increase in tracheal pressure.

Regulatory Respiratory Reflexes

The SARs are excited by lung inflation and suppressed by lung deflation. The RARs are also excited by lung inflation, but their discharge is not sustained (Figure 8–8).

Slowly Adapting Pulmonary Receptors Mediate Vagal Volume Feedback

> SARs are stimulated by each inspiration and fire with a progressively augmenting discharge throughout the duration of an inspiration.

Thus, these mechanoreceptors continuously provide information about lung volume, changes in lung volume, and rate of change in lung volume.

> SAR input is *inhibitory* to P-cells in the DRG and to the I-neurons in the VRG, and *excitatory* to the E-neurons in the caudal VRG.

More than a century ago, Breuer, working in Hering's laboratory, analyzed the reflex responses evoked by this vagal input. Today these reflex responses are called the Breuer-Hering (or Hering-Breuer) reflexes. Because these reflexes are much more easily demonstrated in infants than in adult humans, some deny their physiological significance in adults.

> When *SAR feedback* is intact, lung inflation during an inspiration is prematurely terminated (Figure 8–9).

By counteracting and limiting lung inflation, SAR input sets the *duration* of each inspiration (i.e., inspiratory time, T_I) and is thus a determinant of breathing frequency. Because of this premature termination of inspiration and the facilitation of expiration, SAR feedback controls the end-expiratory lung volume and, hence, the operating length of the diaphragm. In this way SAR feedback keeps the length of the diaphragm in an operating range optimal for keeping ventilatory efficiency maximal and the cost of breathing minimal.

When vagal feedback is eliminated by cutting the vagus nerves, I-neurons are relieved of SAR-initiated inhibition. Consequently, a vagotomized animal breathes very deeply and slowly (Figure 8–9). Despite the fact that expired minute ventilation ($\dot{V}_E$) is essentially unchanged, the deep slow-breathing pattern of the vagotomized animal is inefficient and costly.

Rapidly Adapting Pulmonary Receptors Mediate the Deflation Reflex

Vagal *mechanoreceptors* that are excited by an imposed lung deflation (e.g., during negative pressure breathing) are rapidly adapting (RARs).

Their sensory terminations in the periphery are located in a nerve complex in the columnar cell epithelium of the airway, but the exact structure or physical relationship to the airway smooth muscle is not clear. Vagal afferent fibers of the deflation receptors are myelinated and project to sites in the dorsal NTS that are distinct from those of the SARs. Because the RAR input is *excitatory* to I-neurons

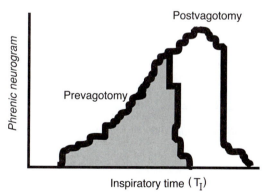

Figure 8–9
Phrenic neurogram (ordinate) before and after vagotomy. The rising slope of the inspiratory discharge is unaffected by vagotomy, but the duration and amplitude increase in the absence of vagal feedback. Normally this feedback activates an inspiratory "off-switch."

and *inhibitory* to E-neurons, its output prevents lung collapse by counteracting lung deflation.

Defense Reflexes Mediated by Irritant Receptors

Another group of RARs in the lungs and airways is served by either non-myelinated pulmonary or bronchial C-fibers, depending on the location and blood supply of the afferent terminals. Selective stimulation of these fibers evokes rapid, shallow breathing; bronchoconstriction; increased airway secretion; and cardiovascular depressor effects (e.g., decrease in heart rate, arterial blood pressure, cardiac output, and cardiac contractility). The pulmonary C-fibers are sensitive to lung inflation and lung congestion, whereas the bronchial afferents are stimulated by humoral mediators of inflammation such as histamine, prosta-glandins, and bradykinins.

> The bronchial RARs have the important function of signaling onset of pathology in the airways.

For example, they become very active in conditions such as pulmonary conges-tion, pneumothorax, embolization, or anaphylaxis. The sensory neurons of these RARs lie in the nodose ganglia, and their central projections terminate in the NTS. Second-order neurons project centrally to the respiratory neurons in the dorso-lateral pons, the DRG, the VRG, the dorsal motor nucleus of X, and to areas in-volved in autonomic control of airway smooth muscle and cardiovascular effectors.

Protective Reflexes Mediated by Irritant Receptors

Other functional groups of RARs mediate protective reflexes such as *cough-ing* and *sneezing*.

> These responses defend the airways against inhaled particles and noxious substances.

These are powerful reflexes that function by clearing the lungs and airways of foreign matter or accumulated mucus.

Cough Reflex The afferent limbs of the cough reflex are in the vagus and supe-rior laryngeal nerves (SLN). Irritant (RARs) and nonmyelinated C-fiber nerve endings are distributed to all parts of the lungs, the tracheobronchial tree (vagal), and larynx (SLN). The targets for the central projections from these airway receptors are the caudal NTS and the central respiratory neurons. The targets for the SLN afferents from the larynx are also the caudal NTS and DRG.

> Cough has three phases: (1) inspiratory, (2) compressive, and (3) expulsive.

The deep inspiration, the first phase, is thought to excite the pulmonary stretch receptors (i.e., SRAs), which induce facilitation of expiratory neurons that mediate the compressive and expulsive phases of the cough.

Sneeze Reflex Sneezing is initiated by stimulation of the nasal mucosa with water, cigarette smoke, or a variety of chemical gases. The receptors remain to be identified, but the afferent fibers course in the trigeminal nerves. The central target is thought to be the pontine respiratory group. Ultimately the sneeze motor pattern involves the BÖTC and the I-neurons and E-neurons of the VRG. As opposed to a cough, during the inspiratory effort of a sneeze there are intermittent pauses and during the expulsive phase air is expired through the nose as well as the mouth.

Expulsive Reflexes and Other Functions of Respiratory Muscles

Respiratory muscles are multifunctional in that they participate in numerous expulsive reflexes such as vomiting, defecation, micturition, and parturition. They are also involved in swallowing, speech, postural control, and cardiovascular regulation. The neural integration by which the same muscles can be involved in such a variety of functions remains a major challenge for future investigators.

ONDINE'S CURSE

Normal breathing is an *automatic* motor behavior. As previously discussed, a *central rhythm generator* (CRG) determines the timing of events in each breathing cycle, and a *central pattern generator* (CPG) determines, on a breath-by-breath basis, which muscles are activated, the sequence in which they are activated, and the level to which they are activated.

> In an occasional individual the ability to breathe automatically fails.

This condition is called *Ondine's Curse,* named for the mythical god Ondine who cursed any mortal who fell in love with a goddess with this respiratory affliction.

While awake a patient with absence of automatic breathing will compensate *voluntarily.* However, during sleep the same individual fails to breathe.

> The fact that individuals can voluntarily compensate for lost respiratory function demonstrates that brain regions higher than the medulla or pons have access to the respiratory motoneurons.

It remains to be determined whether cortical control is exerted directly at the spinal level, the medullary level, or both.

The organization of some of the key components of the automatic respiratory control system are summarized in Figure 8–10.

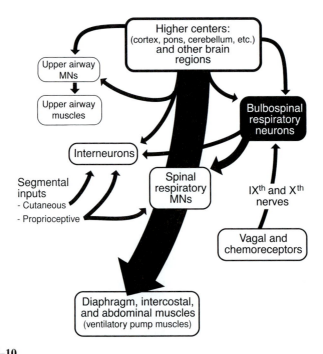

Figure 8–10
Putative neural connections among the many components involved in the control of the respiratory muscles. MN, motoneuron. (Adapted from *Neural Control of the Respiratory Muscles,* A.D. Miller, A.L. Bianchi, and B.P. Bishop, editors. CRC Press, Boca Raton, FL, 1999.)

· C H A P T E R · 9 ·

CORTICAL CONTROL OF VOLUNTARY MOVEMENTS

·

Beverly P. Bishop

Cortical Sources of Descending Motor Commands

Properties of Corticospinal Neurons

Columnar Organization of the Cerebral Cortex

Electrical Recordings from Neurons in the Motor Cortex

Functional Consequences of Damage to the Motor Cortex

· · · · · · · · · · · ·

> *Voluntary movements* are the third and highest hierarchy of motor control. These are planned, learned, skilled, purposeful movements that depend heavily, among other sources, on premotoneurons in the cerebral cortex.

The motor cortex is on the efferent limb of the motor pathway. During the execution of voluntary movements, automatic postural reflexes are required to prepare and support the body's posture throughout the movement. The basal ganglia and cerebellum also play important roles in control of movement through their reciprocal connections with the cortex.

CORTICAL SOURCES OF DESCENDING MOTOR COMMANDS

Neurons in many sites of the cerebral cortex project to the brain stem and spinal cord.

> Because damage to the *primary motor cortex* produces profound motor deficits, its bulbar and spinal projections have received major attention.

The motor cortex lies in the precentral gyrus anterior to the central sulcus (Figure 9–1A). Removal of this region of the cerebral cortex in an infant produces little immediate observable deficit in movement; however, as the infant matures, complex, skilled motor performance never appears. The resulting motor deficits persist throughout the individual's life.

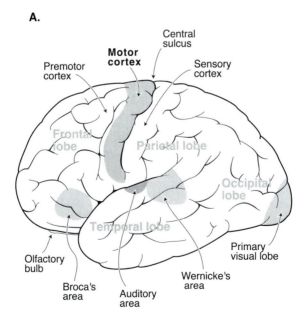

Figure 9–1 (A)
Lateral view of the left cerebral cortex showing the location of the motor cortex.

The *primary motor cortex* is the thickest part of the brain (up to 4.5 mm in the human brain), and, like all other parts of the *cerebral* cortex, is composed of six layers. Neurons within the same layer have similar shapes, patterns of connectivity, and functions. The motor cortex has been subdivided into multiple areas on the basis of its cytoarchitecture and goes by a variety of names including the motor strip, M_1, and Brodmann's areas 4 and 6.

The primary motor cortex is somatotopically organized (Figure 9–1B), that is, it contains an orderly motor map (Wilder Penfield's homunculus) of contralateral body regions to which each cortical region projects.

Different body regions have unequal cortical representation, with regions requiring precise motor control (e.g., the digits and tongue) having the largest representation. In other words, those regions of the body with the greatest density of receptors have the greatest cortical representation or, said in another way, receptors with the smallest receptive fields in the periphery have the greatest cortical representation. Each area of this motor map is thought to control movements, not muscles, of particular body parts.

B.

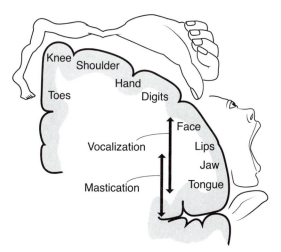

Figure 9–1 (B)
Cortex in coronal section showing the somatotopic organization of the motor area derived from Wilder Penfield's homunculus.

Major Pathways Between the Motor Cortex and the Lower Motoneurons

The *corticobulbar* and *corticospinal pathways* are two descending motor tracts that originate from different regions of the cerebral cortex and terminate in the brain stem and spinal cord, respectively.

These two tracts take similar initial trajectories in that their axons project through the deep layers of the cortex, the internal capsule, and the middle portion of the crus cerebri. The *corticobulbar fibers* originate primarily in the regions of the sensorimotor cortex representing the face. The cell bodies lie in the fifth and sixth cortical layers, and their parent axons terminate in the somatic and brachial efferent nuclei in the brain stem. The axons of the corticospinal tract are gathered together in the basilar pons and decussate (cross) to the contralateral side in the pyramids of the caudal medulla.

The *corticospinal tract* is also known as the *pyramidal tract.*

It originates from 20,000 to 600,000 large neurons (Betz cells) and 580,000 smaller neurons residing in regions of the motor cortex other than the facial area and from cortical areas outside the primary motor cortex (Figure 9–2). The corticospinal tracts are the longest and among the largest tracts of the central nervous system (CNS), having an estimated 10^6 axons.

Beyond the pyramids the corticospinal tract separates into the *lateral* and *ventral corticospinal tracts.*

The *lateral corticospinal pathway* is composed of corticospinal neurons located in the hand and foot areas of the primary motor cortex. These neurons function as private lines by making synapses directly on the spinal motoneurons that innervate the distal muscles controlling the digits. This monosynaptic lateral pathway is the most direct pathway from the cortex to the spinal motoneurons.

The *ventral corticospinal pathway* originates in cortical regions anterior to the motor cortex, and its axons descend to synapse on interneurons in the intermediate gray and among the motor nuclei of the ventromedial ventral horn (Rexed's laminae VII and VIII). Motoneurons in these spinal nuclei innervate the proximal and axial (trunk) muscles.

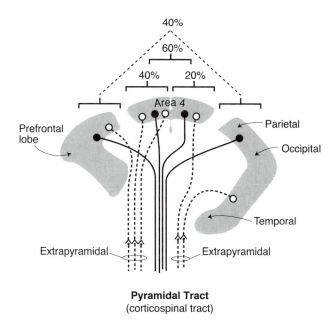

Pyramidal Tract
(corticospinal tract)

Figure 9–2
Cortical regions from which the pyramidal tract originates. Area 4 contributes only 60%, with the prefrontal and parietal lobes contributing the remaining 40% to the pyramidal tract.

PROPERTIES OF CORTICOSPINAL NEURONS

Intrinsic morphological and anatomical characteristics of the so-called upper motoneurons endow them with capabilities that distinguish them very dramatically from the lower motoneurons in the ventral horns of the spinal cord. During development, the cortical neurons that ultimately form the pyramidal tract develop large pyramidal-shaped cell bodies whose diameters range from 10 to 120 μm (Figure 9–3). The apex of the cell body is oriented toward the surface of the cortex.

Dendrites of the premotor cortical neurons increase in size, length, and number with age. This dendritic expansion is an important maturational phenomenon in CNS development.

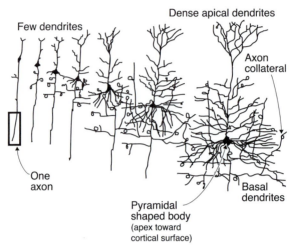

Figure 9–3
Differentiation and maturation of a pyramidal cell. Apical dendrites form at the cortical surface. Basal dendrites form at the cell body's base. Dendritic spines form as projections from dendritic stalks. Axon collaterals (small open circles) terminate within the cortex. Axons project through the internal capsule to form descending tracts.

The dendrites provide large surface areas that can receive both extra- and intracortical inputs. The long *apical dendrites* lie in parallel and are directed toward the surface of the cortex. They expand in great arbors at their termination near the cortical surface. Initially only a few *basal or lateral dendrites* form, but these become pronounced as the cell matures.

Dendrites soon give rise to *dendritic spines.*

The morphological consequence of this expansion of the dendritic structure is an enhanced surface area for synapse formation, the substrate for dense inputs from diverse sources. Sensory feedback, although not essential for initiating or carrying out movements, optimizes and improves (fine-tunes) the efficiency of movements.

Axons of these cortical premotor neurons grow out almost from the moment the parent cell migrates from the germinal layer. The growth cones of the elongating axons make no errors in selecting the sites to which they grow. Axonal growth through the forebrain and brain stem is slow, but speeds up, and occurs in spurts in the dorsal columns.

Axon collaterals, a striking feature of pyramidal neurons, provide the neural substrate for intracortical communication.

Before leaving the cortex the pyramidal cell has given rise to many axon collaterals that terminate in synaptic connections with neurons in the same or more superficial layers of the cortex (Figure 9–3). The parent axon also forms axon collaterals outside the cortex. These make projections to many subcortical nuclei in the brain (Figure 9–4). As a functional consequence of an axon's expansive collateralization, information is projected concurrently to diverse supraspinal and spinal targets. Thus, signals carried by any one premotor cortical neuron diverge to influence a myriad of postsynaptic elements along the length of the neural axis. This neural substrate results in a functional distributed motor map that regulates movements rather than discrete muscle contractions.

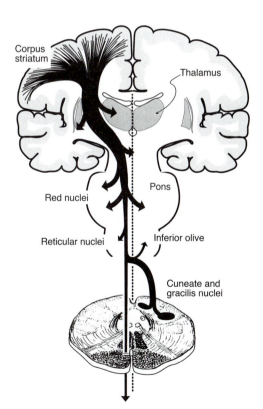

Figure 9–4
Destinations of corticospinal axons. Axon collaterals project to many subcortical sites in their trajectory to their bulbar and spinal destinations.

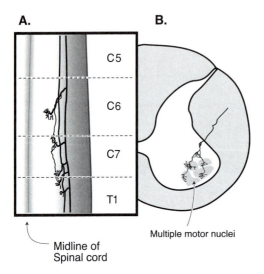

A.

B.

C5

C6

C7

T1

Midline of
Spinal cord

Multiple motor nuclei

Figure 9–5
Spinal terminations of
corticospinal neurons. (**A**)
A single axon may terminate
over several spinal segments.
(**B**) Terminals arborize to
synapse directly and indirectly
on α and γ motoneurons in
multiple synergistic motor
nuclei over a number of spinal
levels.

> Axons project through the internal capsule to form the descending corti-
> cobulbar and corticospinal tracts.

At their spinal destination the descending axons of the pyramidal cells
synapse both directly and indirectly via interneurons on spinal motoneurons span-
ning several spinal segments (Figure 9–5A). A single axon terminates in a mas-
sive terminal arbor permitting synapse formation within several synergistic motor
pools (Figure 9–5B). After synapse formation the axons become heavily myelinated and are therefore rapidly conducting.

COLUMNAR ORGANIZATION
OF THE CEREBRAL CORTEX

> In addition to its layered structure, the cerebral cortex has a *columnar
> organization.*

For example, most of the premotor neurons lying in the same column of the
thumb area of the motor cortex share a similar function. This information was
derived from experiments in which intracortical microstimulation was system-

atically applied at progressively greater depths. As shown by the results in Figure 9–6, stimulation at sites falling on the vertical tract (solid circles) evoked thumb adduction, whereas stimulation on an adjacent tract (solid squares) evoked thumb abduction. These findings and other types of experimental data support the concept that

> individual cortical neurons control movements of small groups of muscles rather than single muscles.

Its topographical, columnar, and layered organization endows the motor cortex with its distinctive functional characteristics.

Additional Descending Pathways Involved in Voluntary Movements

Several descending motor pathways arise from brain regions other than the cerebral cortex. As mentioned previously, premotor cortical neurons send axons,

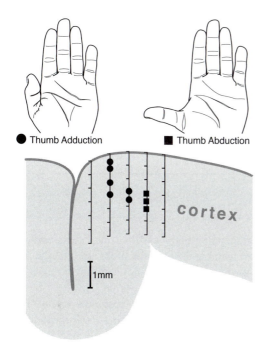

Figure 9–6
Columnar organization of the cortical thumb area. Motor responses evoked by microstimuli applied at different depths from the cortical surface. Stimulation at sites within the same column (vertical lines) evokes similar thumb function (e.g., stimulation at solid circles evoked thumb adduction). Neurons in the same column share similar functions.

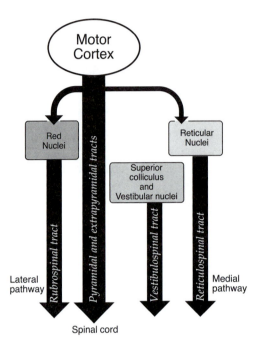

Figure 9–7
Extrapyramidal pathways involved in the control of voluntary movements. Axonal collaterals from descending cortical neurons project to the red nucleus and the reticular nuclei but not to the superior colliculus or the vestibular nuclei. These three nuclei (shown as gray boxes) give rise to lateral and medial descending pathways that control the postural components essential for supporting voluntary movements.

axon collaterals, or both to synapse in the red nucleus and the reticular formation (Figure 9–4 and Figure 9–7).

The *rubrospinal tract* projects from neurons in the red nucleus whose axons, at the level of the pons, cross to the contralateral side and join the lateral pathway (Figure 9–7). Rubrospinal axons, like those of the lateral corticospinal tract, terminate in the dorsolateral spinal cord in the vicinity of the motoneurons controlling the distal muscles of the arm, hand, and fingers. The rubrospinal tract is smaller in humans than in other mammals. Nonetheless, recordings of its activity suggest that

> the *red nucleus* plays a significant role in hand movements.

In monkeys, lesions of the lateral descending pathways (i.e., the lateral corticospinal and the rubrospinal tracts) result in paralysis of the limbs; in time the use of the extremities for climbing and locomotion recover, although finger dexterity never returns.

The vestibulospinal tract arises from neurons in the vestibular nuclei that receive no known direct inputs from the motor cortex (Figure 9–7). Nonetheless, this pathway provides an important input to the ventromedial motor nuclei of the spinal cord.

The *vestibulospinal tract* is essential for controlling posture, especially of the head and neck.

The reticulospinal tract arises from the medial reticular formation of the pons and medulla.

The *reticulospinal tract* is essential for controlling the antigravity muscles and the posture of the trunk.

Neurons in the reticular nuclei are recipients of inputs from the motor cortex (Figure 9–4) and from most sensory systems. Axons of reticular neurons project to the ventromedial spinal nuclei by the medial pathway (Figure 9–7). As would be expected, lesions to any of these ventrally projecting systems disrupt function of both proximal limbs and axial muscles.

Thus, compared with the corticospinal tracts, the noncorticospinal tracts exert less direct control over movements, do not send their axons through the pyramids, and have historically been considered important components of the *extrapyramidal* system (Figure 9–2).

ELECTRICAL RECORDINGS FROM NEURONS IN THE MOTOR CORTEX

Significant information about the role of the motor cortex in voluntary movements has been derived from recording the electrical activity from cortical premotor neurons before and during a performance of a learned movement.

Figure 9–8A shows one of the earliest experimental setups for obtaining such records. Monkeys were trained to perform a wrist flexion and extension to lift different weights. Once trained, the monkey was anesthetized and recording electrodes were implanted in the wrist area of the motor cortex and in the flexor and extensor wrist muscles in the periphery for subsequent recording sessions. An *antidromic test* was used to verify that the cortical recording electrode was detecting activity in a wrist neuron. An action potential initiated by applying a stimulus to an axon evokes a nerve action potential that is conducted both orthodromically and antidromically. In this case the antidromic test was applied to determine whether an electric shock delivered to the pyramidal tract evoked

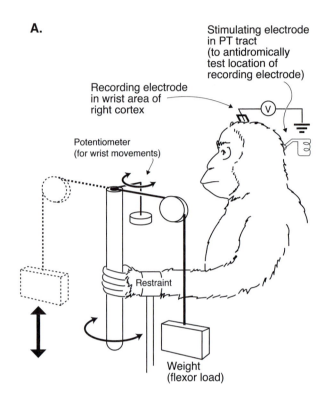

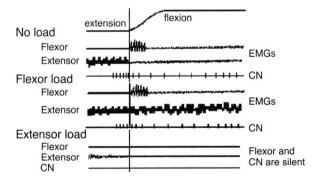

Figure 9–8
(**A**) Experimental setup for obtaining cortical recordings in an awake, performing monkey. (After E.V. Evarts, *J Neurophysiol* 1968;31:14–27). (**B**) Cortical neuron (CN) recording of wrist flexor while animal alternately flexes and extends the wrist. The conclusion is that CN codes for force.

action potentials in both the cortical wrist neuron (excited antidromically) and the wrist muscle (excited orthodromically). Recordings from the awake performing monkey revealed that the cortical wrist flexion neuron was silent during wrist extension but began discharging several hundreds of milliseconds before the occurrence of the actual wrist flexion. During flexion the firing rate of the flexor neuron progressively accelerated, reaching its highest frequency when the resistance (load) was greatest. The cortical wrist extension neuron was silent during flexion but active during extension.

Careful analysis of records acquired during a variety of experimental paradigms revealed that the activity of the cortical wrist neurons varied in relation to a number of mechanical parameters of each wrist movement the monkey performed.

> Among the parameters of movement that have been shown to be coded in the activity of a cortical neuron are *force, change of force, joint position, direction of the movement,* and *velocity of the movement.*

A single cortical neuron may code for one or several of these movement parameters, with most neurons being broadly tuned. Furthermore, any given movement parameter is represented not by one type of cortical neuron but by an ensemble of neurons that may be widely distributed within the topographical map for any particular body part. Individual neurons that fire during a given movement show only coarse tuning to the direction of the movement, but presumably the activity of ensembles of neurons provides precise information.

An important question remains to be answered: What features of the motor system allow neuronal networks to produce flexible outputs? How can the control systems of motor activities deal with a variable environment? Based on findings from a variety of experimental paradigms, it has been shown that

> neuronal circuits are not hard-wired entities, but rather are multifunctional, flexible networks that are reconfigured to produce different outputs under varying conditions.

For example, a cortical neuron that fires when the thumb and index finger are used to pick up a seed does not fire when a ball is grasped. Thus, we see that the activity of a single unit cannot provide answers to questions about how motor output is controlled. Grasping, which has been called the "hallmark of dexterous hands," requires the coding of the size and shape of the object to be grasped and the transformation of these properties into an appropriate pattern of finger and wrist movement. It is known that such a transformation takes place in a neural circuit that is formed by the inferior parietal lobule and the inferior premotor area. It is, however, not known how the transformation takes place.

FUNCTIONAL CONSEQUENCES OF DAMAGE TO THE MOTOR CORTEX

Despite the skull's bony protection of the brain, each year in the United States about 200,000 people sustain severe head injuries and another 400,000 suffer strokes.

Damage to the motor cortex disrupts voluntary movements.

Whether the damage is the result of head injury, stroke, brain tumor, brain cancer, or neurosurgical interventions, a pure pyramidal lesion is rare. Thus, many of the motor disturbances following head injuries, stroke, or other causes are the result of the involvement of both extrapyramidal and corticospinal systems. However, if the corticospinal tracts are selectively lesioned in an experimental animal, the result is loss of muscle tone (flaccid paralysis) and absence of reflexes in the involved parts. Because finger dexterity depends critically on the motor cortex, it is among the motor skills most disturbed by pyramidectomy or any injury to the motor cortex. This motor deficit is profound and permanent. Patients with such a lesion can never again move their fingers individually to tie shoelaces, button buttons, or manually use or manipulate utensils. Voluntary movements require a functioning motor cortex.

· C H A P T E R · 1 0 ·

THE NIGROSTRIATAL AND MESOLIMBIC DOPAMINE TRACTS

·

Elaine M. Hull

The Nigrostriatal and Mesolimbic Tracts

The Nigrostriatal/Basal Ganglia System

The Mesolimbic System

Summary

THE NIGROSTRIATAL AND MESOLIMBIC TRACTS

Anatomy

> Two major *dopaminergic tracts,* ascending in parallel from the midbrain to the heart of the forebrain, are very important for self-initiation of movements and for motivation, respectively.

Cell bodies of the nigrostriatal tract lie in the substantia nigra pars compacta (SNc) of the midbrain, designated A9. These neurons contain neuromelanin, which gives them a black appearance and, therefore, their name. Their axons ascend to the caudate nucleus and putamen (collectively termed the dorsal striatum), which are part of the basal ganglia (Figure 10–1).

Cell bodies of the mesolimbic tract (also referred to as the mesocorticolimbic tract) lie adjacent to the substantia nigra in the ventral tegmental area (VTA, A10); their axons ascend to the nucleus accumbens (ventral striatum), the olfactory tubercle, several limbic structures, and the prefrontal cortex (Figure 10–2).

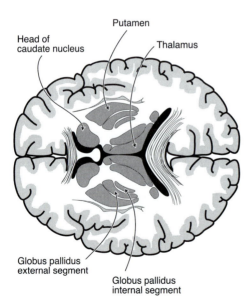

Figure 10–1
Horizontal section of the human brain at the level of the basal ganglia.

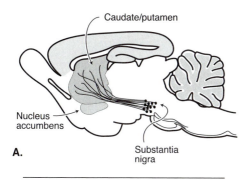

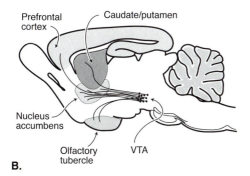

Figure 10–2
Longitudinal sections through the rat brain showing the ascending axons of the nigrostriatal (**A**) and mesolimbic (**B**) dopamine tracts.

THE NIGROSTRIATAL/BASAL GANGLIA SYSTEM

The *nigrostriatal/basal ganglia system* contributes to the triggering of self-initiated movements and to postural adjustments.

It consists of both direct and indirect pathways.

Direct Pathway

The *direct pathway* is a positive feedback loop, by which cortical areas that initiated the activity are further excited.

There are two consecutive inhibitory influences, followed by an excitatory influence (Figure 10–3).

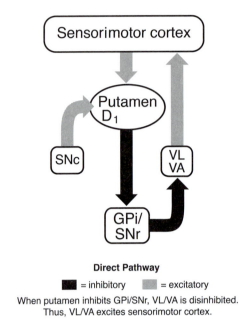

Direct Pathway

■ = inhibitory　　■ = excitatory

When putamen inhibits GPi/SNr, VL/VA is disinhibited.
Thus, VL/VA excites sensorimotor cortex.

Figure 10–3
Nigrostriatal direct pathway.

Stimulating the first inhibitory path (striatum to globus pallidus internal segment, GPi) inhibits the second inhibitory path (GPi to ventrolateral and ventral anterior nuclei of the thalamus, VL/VA), thereby disinhibiting the final excitatory path (thalamus to somatosensory and motor cortex). Therefore, the cortical areas that initiate a movement are able to augment that process via the direct pathway.

Indirect Pathway

The *indirect pathway* is a negative feedback loop.

It, too, begins with two inhibitory paths (striatum to globus pallidus external segment, GPe, and GPe to subthalamic nucleus, STN). This disinhibits an excitatory path (STN to GPi). So far, this is similar to the direct pathway, in that activation of the first inhibitory pathway results in disinhibition of an excitatory pathway. However, this excitatory pathway ends not at the cortex, but on another inhibitory path (GPi to thalamus). Because the thalamus normally excites the cortex, inhibition of the thalamus results in less input to the cortex, thereby inhibiting movement (Figure 10–4).

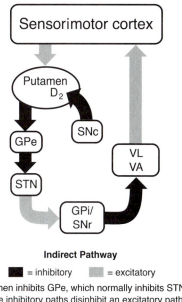

Indirect Pathway

■ = inhibitory   ▨ = excitatory

Putamen inhibits GPe, which normally inhibits STN.
Those inhibitory paths disinhibit an excitatory path.
(STN ---> GPi/SNr)
But that excitatory path ends on another inhibitory path!
(GPi/SNr ---> VL/VA)
Thus, VL/VA can't excite cortex.

Figure 10–4
Nigrostriatal indirect pathway.

It may seem counterintuitive to have opposing direct and indirect pathways. However, they may either sharpen the influence on behavior, much like the sharpening of receptive fields in the visual system, or they may provide greater control over movement, similar to having both inhibitory and excitatory postsynaptic potentials (IPSPs and EPSPs) on the same neuron.

The Role of Dopamine

Dopamine has an excitatory effect on the direct (excitatory) pathway via D_1-like receptors and an inhibitory effect on the indirect (inhibitory) pathway via D_2-like receptors. Thus, both effects increase the output of the system.

In the case of the nigrostriatal/basal ganglia system, dopamine enhances the initiation of movements, and in the case of the mesolimbic system, it increases motivation and/or reward (Figure 10–5).

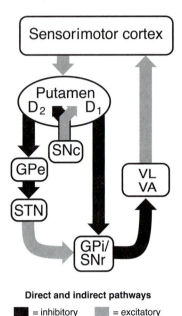

Direct and indirect pathways
■ = inhibitory ▨ = excitatory

Figure 10–5
Both nigrostriatal pathways.

Input to the Nigrostriatal and Mesolimbic Tracts

> Major *excitatory influences* are from the prefrontal cortex to the nucleus accumbens and from the sensorimotor cortex to the dorsal striatum, with glutamate as the transmitter, and from the pedunculopontine nuclei in the pons, with acetylcholine as the transmitter.

Therefore, either the prefrontal or sensorimotor cortex or the pontine reticular formation can activate the direct and indirect pathways. The primary excitatory input to the dopamine cells is from the reticular formation, which responds to any sudden or important stimulus.

> Major *inhibitory inputs* are from GABAergic neurons in the dorsal and ventral striatum and from the dopamine cells themselves, which release dopamine from their dendrites, cell bodies, and axon terminals, all of which contain inhibitory autoreceptors.

Both of these sources of inhibition are therefore negative feedback loops.

Postsynaptic Actions of Dopamine

Dopamine does not directly excite or inhibit postsynaptic neurons. Rather, it alters the voltage sensitivity of voltage-sensitive K^+ channels.

D_1 receptors shift the threshold to a lower membrane voltage, so that the outward flow of K^+ is less likely to occur, and the neuron is more responsive to depolarizing input. With depolarization, the Mg^{2+} block of N-methyl-D-aspartate (NMDA) receptors is removed, and they are therefore more likely to be activated by glutamate. Thus, stimulation of D_1 receptors enables the excitatory influence from the cortex to activate the direct pathway. On the other hand, stimulation of D_2 receptors has the opposite influence, rendering the postsynaptic neurons less excitable. Because D_2 receptors are located primarily on neurons forming the initial segment of the indirect (inhibitory) pathway, dopamine will inhibit that pathway, with a resulting disinhibition of the thalamocortical path.

Therefore, dopamine (via D_1 receptors) *activates* the direct pathway and (via D_2 receptors) *inhibits* the indirect pathway.

Both of these actions result in enhanced ability to initiate movements or increased motivation.

Dopamine in the dorsal and ventral striatum arises from both synaptic and nonsynaptic (axon varicosities) sources. Dopamine diffuses some distance from the site of release, resulting in volume conduction of the neurotransmitter. There are two firing modes of nigrostriatal and mesolimbic neurons: phasic and burst firing. *Phasic release* is directly related to the firing rate of the dopamine neurons. *Burst firing* increases dopamine release exponentially. However, heteroceptors on dopamine terminals modulate dopamine release, either increasing or decreasing the amount of neurotransmitter released in response to action potentials. There is a strong correlation between firing rate and motor activity, and the increases in firing rate frequently anticipate motor activity.

Detection of Dopamine: Methods

Because dopamine diffuses from its site of release, dopamine overflow can be detected by either *microdialysis* or *voltammetry.*

In microdialysis, artificial cerebrospinal fluid is pumped very slowly into a probe, which has a closed "sock" of dialysis membrane attached to the end. Because the end of the membrane is plugged, the fluid must return up a (usually concentric) length of very fine silica tubing, which in turn ends either in a collecting tube or an on-line injector. During the time the fluid is in the dialysis membrane sock, small molecules, such as monoamines and their metabolites, can diffuse from the extracellular fluid into the dialysate. Conversely, drugs can be delivered into the brain from the dialysate. Neurotransmitters and their metabolites can be detected in the dialysate using electrochemical detection. Microdialysis provides an accurate estimate of several neurotransmitters and their metabolites. However, the sampling time is relatively long (usually 3 to 20 min), and the membrane socks are relatively large (210 μm in diameter and 1 to 3 mm in length) (Figure 10–6).

Voltammetry employs carbon fiber electrodes coated with a substance that selectively allows oxidation of dopamine. It has a much shorter sampling time (fractions of seconds) than microdialysis and much finer spatial resolution. However, it does not have complete specificity regarding the molecule being measured and cannot provide assessments of multiple transmitters.

The third major technique for studying dopaminergic influence is single neuron recording of dopamine cell bodies. This technique provides excellent time resolution and a quantitative measure of neuronal activity. However, it does not reflect the spatial distribution of the terminals or the influence of heteroceptors on release.

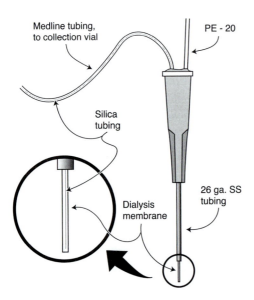

Figure 10–6
Microdialysis probe.

Parkinson Disease

> Degeneration of the nigrostriatal tract results in *Parkinson disease,* which is characterized by tremor at rest, difficulty initiating movements, rigidity, postural instability, and cognitive problems.

Patients frequently lose 80% of the nigrostriatal neurons before symptoms appear. The reason for the late appearance of symptoms is that the dopamine systems are able to compensate for the loss of neurons by increasing synthesis and release of dopamine in the remaining neurons and by increasing postsynaptic receptors. Some cases of Parkinson disease are based on inheritance. However, most appear to be related to environmental toxins, drugs, and trauma, or to unknown factors. Dopamine, itself, can be metabolized to produce free radicals and H_2O_2, which can lead to membrane disruption. Therefore, the increased dopamine synthesis and metabolism in the remaining neurons may actually be toxic for the neurons, leading to a downward spiral of symptoms.

The standard treatment for Parkinson disease is administration of L-dopa, the precursor of dopamine. However, although this alleviates symptoms, it also increases metabolism of dopamine, thereby contributing to the potential toxicity. The dopamine agonist apomorphine has been used with some success. There have been two types of surgical treatments for Parkinson disease. First, tissue from either human fetuses or the patient's own adrenal medulla has been grafted into the caudate nucleus. The patients who benefited most from this procedure were relatively young, with a recent (in several cases, drug-induced) onset of the disease. The other surgical treatment is to make a lesion in the STN or the GPi/substantia nigra pars reticulata (SNr). Because STN excites GPi/SNr, which in turn inhibits the VL/VA nuclei of the thalamus, a lesion of either STN or GPi/SNr would disinhibit the thalamocortical excitation. Strangely enough, stimulation of these structures, via surgically implanted electrodes, has effects similar to those of lesions. However, one possibility is that the stimulation may, in fact, produce a functional lesion.

THE MESOLIMBIC SYSTEM

> The *mesolimbic dopamine tract* parallels the nigrostriatal dopamine tract.

It begins in the VTA of the midbrain, adjacent to the substantia nigra, and ends in the nucleus accumbens (NAcc), or ventral striatum. It also has terminals in the olfactory tubercle, in several limbic system structures (amygdala, lateral septum, and bed nucleus of the stria terminalis), as well as in the prefrontal cortex. This chapter will focus primarily on the terminals in the NAcc, because most of the research on the mesolimbic tract has been similarly focused.

> Whereas the nigrostriatal tract primarily facilitates self-initiated movements, the *mesolimbic tract* increases responsiveness to internal and external stimuli and promotes motivation for numerous goals.

It may also contribute to the sense of reward after achieving those goals. This tract also plays a role in drug addiction and schizophrenia.

Direct Pathway

> The *direct pathway* in the mesolimbic system begins in the NAcc, which in turn inhibits the ventral pallidum.

This results in disinhibition of the mediodorsal (MD) thalamus of the thalamus, which excites the prefrontal cortex (PFC). Thus, in both the nigrostriatal and mesolimbic systems, stimulation of the direct pathway results in excitation of the sensorimotor or prefrontal cortex. Although the relative distributions of the D_1 and D_2 families of receptors in the direct and indirect pathways have been investigated less thoroughly in the mesolimbic system than in the nigrostriatal system, similar patterns of distribution in the two systems have been reported. Furthermore, the known properties of the D_1 receptor suggest that it may play a similar role in the two systems (Figure 10–7).

Indirect Pathway

> The *indirect pathway* is, again, a negative feedback loop.

It, too, begins with two inhibitory paths [NAcc to ventral pallidum (VP), and VP to STN]. This disinhibits an excitatory path (STN back to VP). Thus, activation of the first inhibitory pathway results in disinhibition of an excitatory path-

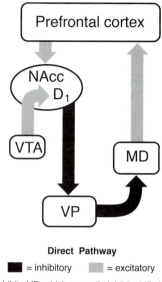

Direct Pathway

■ = inhibitory ▨ = excitatory

NAcc inhibits VP, which normally inhibits MD thalamus. Therefore, MD is now disinhibited. MD excites PFC.

Figure 10–7
The direct pathway of the mesolimbic tract.

way. However, this excitatory pathway ends on another inhibitory path [VP to mediodorsal (MD) thalamus]. Because the thalamus normally excites the cortex, inhibition of the thalamus results in less input to the cortex, thereby inhibiting motivation. The dopamine receptors on the first inhibitory tract of the indirect pathway are probably of the D_2 subtype. Because these receptors shift the threshold for the voltage-gated K^+ channels to a less polarized level, the outward flow of K^+ will counter depolarizing influences, and therefore tend to inhibit the postsynaptic cells. Thus, stimulation of D_2 receptors in the NAcc will inhibit the indirect pathway, thereby removing a negative feedback loop. Because stimulation of D_1 receptors facilitates the excitatory direct pathway, and stimulation of D_2 receptors tends to inhibit the inhibitory indirect pathway, both actions of dopamine will enhance the excitatory input from the mediodorsal thalamus to the prefrontal cortex (Figures 10–8 and 10–9).

The nucleus accumbens is divided into a core and a ventromedial "shell" region. The core appears to be more concerned with the motoric expression of motivation, whereas the shell is considered to be part of the extended amygdala (a major limbic system structure) and is important for the acquisition of incentive learning and for primary reward (Figure 10–10).

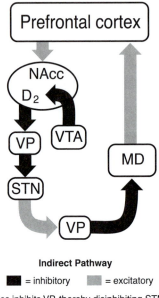

Indirect Pathway

■ = inhibitory   ■ = excitatory

NAcc inhibits VP, thereby disinhibiting STN.
STN now excites VP, but VP inhibits MD.
Therefore, less excitation of PFC.

Figure 10–8
The indirect pathway of the
mesolimbic tract.

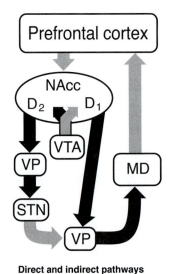

Direct and indirect pathways

■ = inhibitory   ■ = excitatory

Figure 10–9
Both mesolimbic pathways.

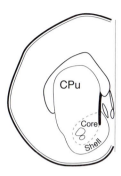

Figure 10–10
Coronal view of the rat brain at the level of the NAcc. CPu, caudate putamen.

The Role of Dopamine in Goal-Directed Behaviors

> Dopamine is thought to increase responsiveness to both external and internal stimuli.

It may also contribute to reward. If dopamine is the major transmitter mediating reward processes, the firing rate of dopaminergic neurons should increase after food or drug delivery and decrease before the next response. This is, indeed, the pattern observed during the first several reinforcements (Figure 10–11A). Similarly, dopamine levels are elevated within a couple of minutes after application of tail pinch, showing that dopamine is also released in response to aversive stimuli and stress (Figure 10–11B). However, after an animal learns to bar press for a reward, dopamine neurons begin to increase their firing rate before the bar press and actually decrease firing when the reward is delivered (Figure 10–12). These data suggest that dopamine is more important for the behavioral activation that secures the goal (or avoidance of aversive stimuli) than for mediation of the reward itself. Consistent with this hypothesis, it has been reported that both nigrostriatal and mesolimbic neurons fire in response to novel attention-grabbing stimuli within almost any stimulus modality. This dopaminergic activity would arouse the motivational fervor of an animal to respond to whatever stimulus is appropriate at the moment. It may also signal the unpredictability of a stimulus and may lead to permanent changes in the dorsal and ventral striatum.

On the other hand,

> dopamine may also mediate important aspects of reward.

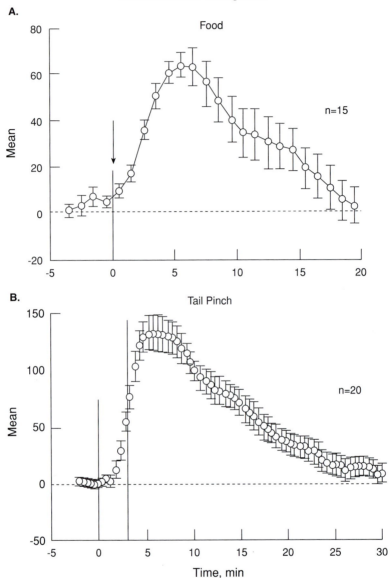

Electrochemical Change, nM

A. Food

n=15

B. Tail Pinch

n=20

Time, min

Figure 10–11
Dopamine levels in the nucleus accumbens of rats, measured with in vivo voltammetry.
(**A**) Dopamine levels before and after presentation of food. (**B**) Dopamine levels before,
during (between vertical lines), and after tail pinch. In both cases, dopamine levels
begin to rise within 2 min of presentation of the stimulus. (From E.A. Kiyatkin, *Neurosci
Biobehav Rev* 1995; 19:573.)

200

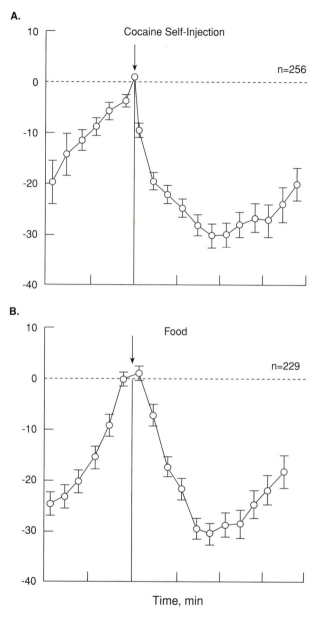

Figure 10–12

Dopamine levels in the nucleus accumbens of rats that have been trained to bar press for cocaine or food. Dopamine levels rise until the bar press, after which they decline. Vertical lines represent the time of the bar press; dashed lines indicate dopamine levels at the time of the previous bar press. (From E.A. Kiyatkin, *Neurosci Biobehav Rev* 1995; 19:573.)

201

All classes of abused drugs increase extracellular dopamine in the NAcc via diverse mechanisms. They also decrease the threshold for electrical brain stimulation reward (i.e., make it easier for the rewarding effect to occur). Conversely, dopamine antagonists, microinjected into the NAcc, decrease brain stimulation reward. Finally, microdialysis shows an increase in dopamine in the NAcc during exposure of a male rat to an estrous female and a further increase during copulation. Thus, dopamine is released during both the appetitive and consummatory (or rewarding) aspects of behavior. Therefore, dopamine may play a role in both the motor activation required to achieve a goal and in the reward itself.

We have seen that dopamine neurons fire before and/or after numerous types of motivated behavior. Is the system able to discriminate among the types of behavior and/or the types of reward? Neurons in the NAcc and prefrontal cortex have been recorded during sessions in which rats self-administered either cocaine or heroin. Very different patterns and timing of activity have been observed, both within and across neurons, as motivational state and incentive or rewarding stimuli were changed. In some cases neurons fired during presentation of stimuli predictive of reward, and in other cases they fired during presentation of the reward itself. Because the firing of dopaminergic neurons appears to be similar across different motivational states, the discriminative nature of NAcc responses suggests that some specificity is conferred by input from the cortex to the NAcc. Thus, dopamine appears to be generally enabling of responses to gain a reward and of the reward itself. On the other hand, the postsynaptic neurons in the NAcc are able to discriminate among rewards and among different phases of conditioning. Similarly, dopamine in the nigrostriatal tract does not carry specific information about motor patterns, but rather enables the cortex to plan and initiate those patterns.

The Role of the Mesolimbic Dopamine System in Drug Addiction

> Mesolimbic dopamine is also important in drug addiction.

Acute administration of cocaine, amphetamine, morphine, ethyl alcohol, and nicotine all increase extracellular dopamine in the NAcc. These drugs also facilitate intracranial electrical self-stimulation (rewarding electrical stimulation of the brain) via dopaminergic mechanisms. Finally, withdrawal from various abused drugs results in decreased extracellular concentrations of dopamine in the NAcc and increased reward threshold.

Numerous cellular changes result from chronic drug administration. These include increased tyrosine hydroxylase (TH, the rate-limiting enzyme in dopamine synthesis) in the VTA (resulting in more dopamine to stimulate autoreceptors on dendrites and cell bodies and therefore decreased firing rate and decreased dopamine release at the terminals in NAcc) and decreased TH in the terminals in the NAcc. The decrease in TH in the NAcc may result from decreased neurofilaments in dopaminergic axons and therefore decreased axonal transport (Figure 10–13).

> Together, these findings suggest that the release of dopamine in the NAcc may produce the rewarding effects of abused drugs and that the decrease in dopamine during drug withdrawal produces the dysphoria characteristic of that state. However, things are not as simple as that.

First, self-administration of opiates is not blocked by dopamine antagonists, suggesting that nondopaminergic synapses mediate opiate reward. However, conditioned place preference for opiates is blocked by dopamine antagonists. In conditioned place preference, an animal is injected with either a drug or saline as

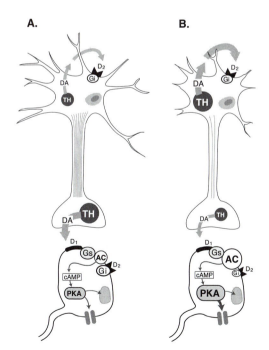

Figure 10–13
(**A**) A schematic drawing of a normal VTA dopamine neuron and a postsynaptic neuron in the nucleus accumbens. (**B**) A schematic drawing of a dopamine neuron and a postsynaptic neuron in a drug-addicted animal. (From E.J. Nestler, *Neuroscientist* 1995;1:212.)

a control. It is then placed into one of two distinctive boxes; drug injections are always followed by placement into one box and saline injections are always followed by placement into the other. After a number of such pairings, the animal is tested in a drug-free state. It is placed into an alley that connects the two boxes and chooses which box to spend more time in. Drugs of abuse, including opiates, reliably result in a greater choice of the box previously associated with drug injections, and this is blocked by dopamine antagonists administered before each drug injection. Therefore, dopamine may be important for the learning of drug–stimulus (the correct box) associations for most abused drugs, although it may mediate the self-administration only of psychostimulants (amphetamine and cocaine), which are indirect dopamine agonists.

A second problem with the dopamine hypothesis of drug withdrawal is that the state of decreased dopamine release during withdrawal should impair all types of motivation, including that for more drug. It is true that motivation for conventional reinforcers is diminished during withdrawal and that the threshold for rewarding electrical brain stimulation is raised (requiring more intense stimulation to elicit reward). However, there is actually an intense craving for drugs. It has been proposed that the difference between conventional reinforcers and abused drugs is that dopaminergic and behavioral responsiveness to conventional reinforcers becomes satiated, whereas drugs short-circuit the neural chain that produces the satiation. This may reinforce the learning of drug–stimulus associations, at the expense of conventional reinforcers.

> It has been suggested that the drug craving may be increased by activation of D_2 receptors in the NAcc and decreased by activation of D_1 receptors there.

In an experiment rats were trained to press a lever to deliver intravenous cocaine in a daily 4-hour schedule. For the first 2 hours cocaine was freely available; during the second 2 hours, saline was substituted. During the saline phase, responding decreased (extinction) (Figure 10–14).

After the decrease in responding, animals were given injections of either a D_1- or a D_2-like agonist to determine whether these drugs would reinstate responding for the saline intravenous infusions. The D_2-like agonist did result in large increases in responding. Therefore, stimulation of D_2-like receptors triggered a relapse (induced craving). The D_1-like agonist did not increase responding at all. Therefore, D_1-like receptors are not implicated in producing craving. Next, the D_1- or D_2-like agonists were given during the saline phase 30 min before an intravenous injection of cocaine to determine whether these agonists would increase or decrease the response to cocaine (Figure 10–15).

The D_2-like agonist greatly increased the responses following the cocaine priming dose. However, the D_1-like agonist completely blocked responding following the cocaine primer. Therefore, the D_1-like agonist not only did not elicit responses, it actually decreased the effectiveness of cocaine.

In other experiments, both D_1- and D_2-like agonists were self-administered by rats and therefore produced rewarding effects of their own. Therefore, the inhibitory effects of the D_1-like agonists on cocaine self-administration were not accompanied by an inhibition of reward. This is especially interesting, because such agonists could be used to treat cocaine addiction. Dopamine antagonists have previously been proposed as possible treatments for cocaine abuse, because they can block the rewarding effects of psychostimulants; however, these antagonists exacerbate withdrawal symptoms and are aversive to both rats and humans. Therefore a better treatment for drug abuse may be D_1-like agonists, which produce rewarding effects of their own but decrease the craving for cocaine.

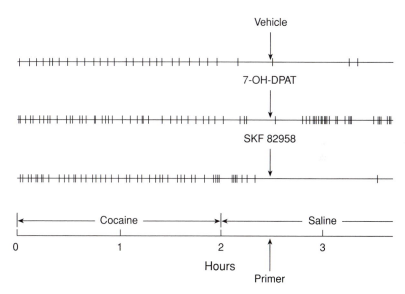

Figure 10–14
Effects of intraperitoneal priming injection with vehicle (saline), the D_2-like dopamine agonist 7-hydroxy-di-n-propylaminotetraline (7-OH-DPAT, 3 mg/kg), or the D_1-like agonist SKF 82958 (1 mg/kg) on reinstatement of nonreinforced lever-press responding in a representative animal. Priming injections were given after extinction from 2 hours of intravenous cocaine self-administration, when only intravenous injections were available. Hatchmarks denote the times of each self-infusion of cocaine in the cocaine phase and of saline in the saline phase. (From D.W. Self et al., *Science* 1996;271:1586.)

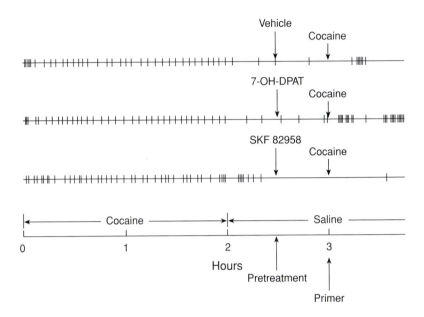

Figure 10–15

Effects of subcutaneous pretreatments with the drug vehicle, the D_2-like dopamine agonist 7-hydroxy-di-*n*-propylaminotetraline (7-OH-DPAT, 0.3 mg/kg), or the D_1-like agonist SKF 82958 (1 mg/kg) on the ability of a low intravenous priming dose of cocaine (2 mg/kg) to reinstate nonreinforced lever-press responding in a representative animal. Priming injections of cocaine were given 30 min after pretreatment with the dopamine receptor agonists during the saline phase of the reinstatement paradigm. Hatchmarks denote the times of each self-infusion of cocaine in the cocaine phase and of saline in the saline phase. (From D.W. Self et al., *Science* 1996;271:1586.)

The Role of the Mesolimbic Dopamine System in Schizophrenia

> Symptoms of *schizophrenia* are divided into two groups: positive symptoms and negative symptoms.

Positive symptoms (characteristics that are abnormal in their presence) include hallucinations, delusions, and thought disorder (consecutive thoughts that have little relationship to one another). Negative symptoms (characteristics that are abnormal in their absence) include flat affect and social withdrawal.

> Numerous brain abnormalities are characteristic of schizophrenia.

Brain volume is decreased, particularly in cortical gray matter, amygdala, hippocampus, and thalamus. Conversely, the lateral and third ventricles are increased in volume (signifying decreased brain tissue). In addition, an abnormal orientation of neurons has been observed in the hippocampus and the surrounding entorhinal cortex. Finally, inappropriate expression of various peptides has been reported.

In spite of the multiple brain abnormalities in schizophrenia, a single hypothesis has dominated much of the thinking about its cause.

> The dopamine hypothesis of schizophrenia proposes that increased levels of, or receptors for, dopamine in the dorsal and/or ventral striatum underlie the disorder.

The primary evidence for this hypothesis is that dopamine antagonists are used to treat psychotic symptoms, whereas dopamine agonists induce or exacerbate such symptoms.

However, there are several problems with the dopamine hypothesis. First, there are different time courses of the effects of antipsychotics on symptoms of schizophrenia compared with those on dopamine synapses. It takes approximately 2 weeks for these drugs to improve symptoms of schizophrenia; however, the drugs block dopamine receptors almost immediately. Second, most typical antipsychotics are more effective in treating positive than negative symptoms. However, some atypical antipsychotics are reported to relieve negative as well as positive symptoms. Third, there is no evidence for increased dopamine levels in the brains of schizophrenics, although there may be increased D_3 receptors in the NAcc. Fourth, there are widespread anatomical abnormalities, including disarrayed neurons in the hippocampus, larger ventricles, and lighter brain weights. It is not clear how alterations of dopamine could affect brain anatomy.

> A recent, more integrative hypothesis proposes that the anatomical abnormalities in schizophrenics reflect deficiencies in neural processing that provide input to the ventral striatum.

Specifically, hallucinations and delusions may result from excessive activity in the hippocampus and surrounding temporal neocortex. These may be assigned undue emotional relevance, due to overactivity in the extended amygdala. Because the prefrontal cortex is hypoactive, it is unable to evaluate and inhibit these excesses. As a result, the ventral striatum is bombarded with incoherent sensory and motivational inputs. In support of this theory, medications that ameliorate the positive symptoms of schizophrenia result in modulation of DNA transcription in the shell of the NAcc, where inputs from the amygdala and the prefrontal and temporal cortices converge. Furthermore, postmortem, neuropsychological, and neuroimaging studies have revealed hyperactivity of the temporal cortex, associated with reality distortion, and hypoactivity of the prefrontal cortex, associated with negative symptoms and poor impulse control.

SUMMARY

In both the nigrostriatal and mesolimbic dopamine systems, dopaminergic activity increases activity in thalamocortical positive feedback pathways. Dopaminergic activity in the nigrostriatal system enhances the ability of the sensorimotor cortex to initiate movements. Degeneration of this tract in Parkinson disease results in impairment of self-initiated movements, among other symptoms. Dopamine in the mesolimbic system promotes behavioral responsiveness to many motivational stimuli and may also mediate or enhance the rewarding characteristics of those stimuli. Dopamine is released following unexpected rewarding stimuli, such as food and psychoactive drugs, or aversive stimuli, or leading up to responses to obtain rewarding stimuli. Drugs of abuse typically increase extracellular levels of dopamine in the mesolimbic system, either directly or indirectly. Furthermore, drug addiction is characterized by decreased dopamine release from mesolimbic neurons, which may promote a state of dysphoria. Finally, excess stimulation of D_3 dopamine receptors in the mesolimbic system, coupled with hypoactivity of the frontal cortex, may contribute to schizophrenia, specifically to a hyperresponsiveness to thoughts or stimuli that give rise to hallucinations or thought disorder.

· C   H   A   P   T   E   R   · 1 1 ·

VISUAL CORTEX: INFORMATION PROCESSING AND DEVELOPMENT

·

Susan B. Udin

Overview and Definitions

The Pathway from the Eye to the Cortex

Decussation

The Lateral Geniculate Nucleus

Striate (Primary Visual) Cortex

Columnar Organization of the Striate Cortex

Ocular Dominance and Binocular Processing

Development of Binocular Connections

Development of Ocular Dominance Columns

Beyond the Striate Cortex

·   ·   ·   ·   ·   ·   ·   ·   ·   ·   ·

OVERVIEW AND DEFINITIONS

STRIATE CORTEX

1. Relatively few center-surround cells.
2. Most cells respond best to straight lines or edges.
3. Some cells respond best to colored objects.
4. Information from the two eyes is combined to make binocular cells.

EXTRASTRIATE CORTEX

1. Striate cortex provides direct or indirect input to dozens of other cortical areas.
2. The *what* stream: some areas are specialized to deal with the shape, form, and identity of objects.
3. The *where* stream: some areas are specialized to deal with the location or movement of objects.

How is information from the retina used by the central nervous system for functions such as perception of form, movement, color, and distance? We will look at three aspects of organization: (1) the columnar organization of the cortex, (2) the parcellation of the cortex into ocular dominance regions, and (3) receptive field organization based on orientation selectivity.

We will focus on processing at the first stage in the cortex, the striate cortex (also known as V1, area 17, or the primary visual cortex).

THE PATHWAY FROM THE EYE TO THE CORTEX

Retinal ganglion cells project to the lateral geniculate nucleus, and cells in the lateral geniculate nucleus project to the striate cortex.

The output of the retina is the retinal ganglion cell axons. There is a *retinotopic* projection to the lateral geniculate nucleus: neighboring cells in the retina project to neighboring cells in the lateral geniculate (Figure 11–1).

DECUSSATION

The *visual field* is the region of space that an eye can see when it is in a particular position. Within the visual field the *receptive field* of a neuron is the location at which a change in visual stimulus causes a change in the electrical state of the neuron.

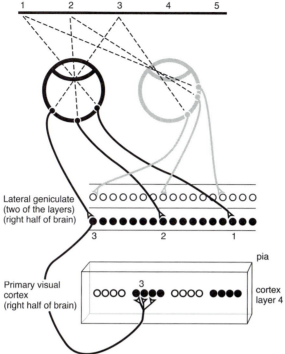

Figure 11–1
Retinogeniculocortical projections. In this schematic, the eyes are shown with the foveas "looking at" position 3 on a screen. Positions 1, 2, and 3 are imaged onto the right halves of the retinas. Ganglion cells in the corresponding regions project to the lateral geniculate nucleus on the right side of the brain; two of the six layers are shown. Cells in the lateral geniculate project to the primary visual cortex on the same side of the brain.

The left half of each retina *sees* the right half of the visual field and transmits that information to the left half of the brain. Information about the left half of the visual field is sent to the right half of the brain.

THE LATERAL GENICULATE NUCLEUS

The *lateral geniculate* has six major layers. Three layers receive input from the left eye and the other three layers receive input from the right eye.

Geniculate cells are monocular.

Different types of retinal ganglion cells project to different geniculate layers: two layers are termed *magnocellular* (large cell) and four layers are termed *parvocellular* (small cell). Most of the input to the two magnocellular layers is from ganglion cells that respond transiently to visual stimuli and that are not very selective for different colors. Each of the two layers gets input from only one eye. Most of the input to the four parvocellular layers is from ganglion cells that respond in a sustained way to visual stimuli and that respond best to particular combinations of colors. Each retina projects to two parvocellular layers.

Geniculate receptive fields are not very different from retinal ganglion cells in receptive field size or overall properties. Cells with foveal receptive fields can be as small as one degree or less; receptive field sizes are larger for cells with more peripheral fields. Almost all geniculate cells have center-surround receptive field organization. They produce little response to diffuse illumination and respond best to small spots of light or dark.

STRIATE (PRIMARY VISUAL) CORTEX

> The striate cortex is a layered structure. Cells in the middle layers of the cortex have a center-surround receptive field, whereas most cells in the other layers have simple or complex receptive fields and respond best to lines or edges. Some cells in all layers respond best to particular distributions of color.

The lateral geniculate projects to the striate cortex (also known as the primary visual cortex or area 17).

The striate cortex is part of the convoluted cortical sheet, which is about 2 mm thick in humans. It has six layers, but the term *layer* in the cortex does not mean the same thing as *layer* when referring to the lateral geniculate.

> In the lateral geniculate, there are very few connections between cells in different layers, whereas in the striate cortex, the cells in the different layers are highly interconnected, and information processing in the cortex depends on these interconnections.

The cortical layers are numbered from 1, at the pial surface, to 6, adjacent to the white matter. Each layer has a distinct set of inputs and outputs that distinguishes it from every other layer.

The lateral geniculate axons project mostly to layer 4C. (Layer 4 has several sublayers, each with particular characteristics of inputs and outputs.) Most of the input to the other layers is relayed from the layer 4 cells. Cells in layer 4C have receptive fields very much like those in the lateral geniculate. The stimuli that activate them best are light or dark spots (center-surround organization). Most cells such as these have monocular receptive fields; in other words, they receive excitation relayed from one eye via the lateral geniculate and do not respond to stimuli presented to the other eye. About half of these cells respond to the left eye and half to the right eye.

The cells in the other layers have very different properties: most respond best to lines and edges rather than spots. These cells are classified as *simple* and *complex.*

Simple Cells

Simple cells are cells in the striate cortex that, unlike those in the ganglion cell layer of the retina or in the lateral geniculate, respond poorly to simple spots or annuli.

A spot in one place evokes a few action potentials, as if in the center of a concentric receptive field. A spot moved to one side evokes no action potentials, as if in the opponent surround. A big spot evokes no action potentials, as if activating both center and surround. However, all of these responses are rather feeble (Figure 11–2).

Substituting a long bar in place of the spot evokes excellent responses, but only for a limited range of orientations per cell (about ± 10°). Some cells prefer a dark bar on a light background, whereas others prefer a light bar on a dark background. Some cells respond best to wide bars and others to narrow bars. Still other cells respond best to a single edge.

The location of the stimulus is crucial; move it one way or the other and it will impinge on the antagonist flank.

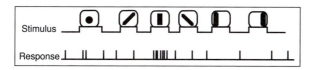

Figure 11–2
Responses of a simple cortical cell. This cell's preferred stimulus orientation is vertical. The cell has a slow spontaneous rate of firing that is increased slightly by the spot near the center of the receptive field; the firing increases sharply when a vertical bar is located in the center of the receptive field but decreases when the same bar is shifted to the left or right. Different orientations of stimuli will activate other cells.

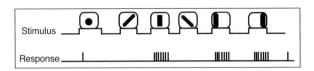

Figure 11–3
A complex cell with a vertical orientation preference can respond to the stimulus anywhere within the receptive field.

Complex Cells

Complex cells are found primarily in layers 2, 3, 5, and 6.

> Like simple cells, *complex cells* also prefer oriented stimuli, but the requirement that the stimulus be in one exact location is less stringent.

There are no obvious inhibitory flanks (Figure 11–3).

Color Cells

Some cells have center-surround receptive fields and are particularly sensitive to specific distributions of color. For instance, some respond best to a red spot on a green background or vice versa, and some respond best to blue/yellow contrasts.

COLUMNAR ORGANIZATION OF THE STRIATE CORTEX

> The cortex is organized into columns that extend from the white matter to the pia and are about 30–100 μm wide.
>
> Almost all the cells in a column have essentially the same preference orientation and the same receptive field center.
>
> The receptive field sizes within a column vary widely.
>
> Each column contains both simple and complex cells.

Orientation Columns

Moving from one column to the adjacent column, the main difference usually is that the cells in the new column respond best to a slightly different stimulus orientation.

About 20 columns are generally found in 1–2 mm of cortex, representing, as a whole, all orientations. One thing that the cells in each column (other than in layer 4C) have in common is that they have very similar receptive field orientations. For each location in the visual field, there is a set of columns containing thousands of cells. At any given time, only a few, or even none, of those cells will be activated; cells become activated only when an object of the correct location, correct orientation, and correct contrast is present.

Each of these arrays of columns includes one or two columns in which most of the cells have center-surround receptive fields and respond best to particular color combinations (Figure 11–4).

Pinwheels

What is the global organization of these columns? Using optical imaging, it is possible to assess how the cells in large numbers of columns respond to different stimuli. When a group of cells is particularly active, the blood supply to these cells increases, and the resulting changes in the reflectiveness of tissue as seen from the surface of the living brain can be monitored optically. The organization forms a *pinwheel* with 360 degrees of orientation surrounding a zone of non-oriented cells.

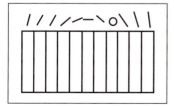

Figure 11–4
A schematic view of a cross-section of the striate cortex. The line above each column shows the preferred orientation for the cells within that column. The circle shows a column with color-selective cells.

Mechanisms to Construct Simple and Complex Receptive Fields

Simple Cells

> Layer 4 cells with center-surround receptive fields that are located along a straight line activate other cortical cells and establish crudely selective oriented receptive fields. Intracortical connections, both excitatory and inhibitory, fine tune the selectivity.

Convergence of inputs with center-surround receptive fields located along a line could excite a simple cell (Figure 11–5).

This circuitry is the basis for orientation selectivity, but experiments in cats indicate that these inputs are not sufficient to account for precision of selectivity; they lead to only about 45-degree tuning. Intracortical circuits are crucial; they provide the majority of synaptic input, both excitatory and inhibitory, to other cortical cells. Many nearby cells provide excitatory input. Other cells, including those at greater distances, provide inhibitory output.

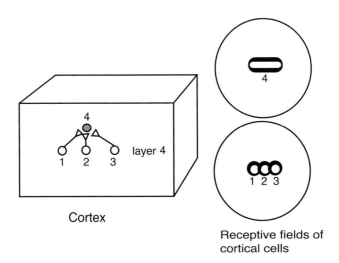

Figure 11–5
If the three cells (1–3) with center-surround receptive fields aligned in a horizontal row converge on cell 4, then cell 4 will respond to a horizontal bright bar at the appropriate position.

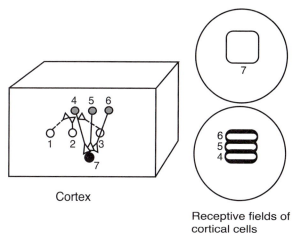

Cortex

Receptive fields of cortical cells

Figure 11–6
Convergence of simple cells 4, 5, and 6 onto cell 7 establishes the complex cell properties that allow cell 7 to respond to a horizontal bright bar anywhere within its receptive field.

Complex Cells

> Intracortical connections from simple cells with slightly displaced receptive field centers converge onto *complex cells* (Figure 11–6).

Some complex cells respond particularly well to moving stimuli. Directionally selective complex cells respond vigorously to a stimulus moving in one direction but not to a stimulus moving in the opposite direction.

OCULAR DOMINANCE AND BINOCULAR PROCESSING

> *Binocular cells:* cells that respond to inputs from both eyes.
>
> *Ocular dominance:* unequal strength of response to input from each of the two eyes.
>
> **HYPERCOLUMN**
> A section of cortex about 2 mm wide.
>
> Contains two ocular dominance zones, one for each eye.
>
> Contains 20 orientation columns, covering 360°.

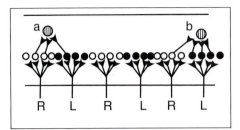

Figure 11–7
Schematic view of the cortex showing that monocular cells in layer 4 of the cortex can strongly activate other cells in the same columns and also activate some cells in other columns.

Binocular Signals

Convergent connections bring input relayed from the left-eye and right-eye layers of the geniculate to cells in the cortex (Figure 11–7).

Most cells, particularly outside of layer 4, respond to input from either eye, but usually the response is stronger from either one eye or the other eye (ocular dominance). Some cells are activated by only the left eye or only the right eye and some are activated by both eyes equally, but most are activated by both eyes, with one eye contributing more than the other (Figure 11–8).

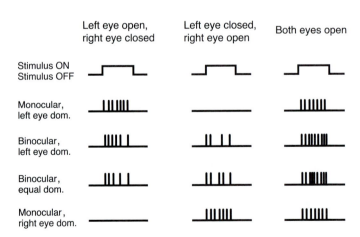

Figure 11–8
The degree of ocular dominance of different cells spans the range from complete domination by one eye (monocularity) to partial domination by one eye to equal representation.

Ocular Dominance Bands

The cortex is organized into ocular dominance domains.

One way to reveal these territories is to use transneuronal transport of a radioactive amino acid. If tritiated proline is injected into one eye, it will be incorporated into protein and transported to the lateral geniculate. During the next few weeks, much of the radioactive protein will be released by the retinogeniculate axons and picked up by the geniculate cells, which then transport it to the cortex. It accumulates in layer 4. The brain can be removed and sections can be cut and coated with photographic emulsion. The radioactive regions will activate the emulsion, which is then developed.

The brain is cut perpendicularly to reveal the depth of the bands (Figure 11–9, top). Note that the bands show up only in the middle layers. Cells in the other layers express ocular dominance because they receive input from those middle layers. Most of the connections are within a column, so most cells above or below a left-eye zone in layer 4 will also be dominated by the left eye.

A tangential slice through layer 4 reveals a zebra-stripe pattern (Figure 11–9). In humans, each stripe is about 1–2 mm wide. Imaging the surface of the brain in awake animals shows the same pattern.

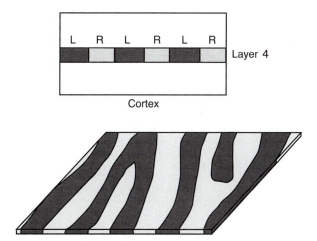

Figure 11–9
Top: Transverse section through the cortex, showing axons from the left-eye and right-eye layers of the lateral geniculate nucleus terminating in separate zones of layer 4. Bottom: Tangential view of layer 4, showing the zebra-stripe pattern of ocular dominance zones.

How do these ocular dominance columns relate to the orientation columns? Ocular dominance columns are about 10 times larger (about 1 mm) than orientation columns (0.1 mm). Each cortical cell located in an orientation column is also located in a larger ocular dominance column. There is no simple geometric relationship between the two systems.

DEVELOPMENT OF BINOCULAR CONNECTIONS

The visual system begins to develop prenatally, and visual experience during infancy and early childhood is essential for normal maturation of the visual cortex. Blockade of vision in one eye (monocular deprivation), if not corrected in the first few months after birth, can lead to permanent loss of visual capabilities.

Critical Period

The orderly division of cortex into left-eye and right-eye regions, with a nearly 50–50 split, requires normal activity during development. Early monocular deprivation can produce irreversible loss of visual function.

Children born with a cataract in one eye must have the cataract removed within the first few months of life or they will have little or no visual function in the affected eye.

There is a *critical period* for this effect. The developing visual system can be permanently altered by visual deprivation during the first few months of life. In contrast, the adult visual system is resistant to such deprivation: a cataract that develops in an adult may block light coming into the eye for years, but when it is removed, vision is immediately restored.

DEVELOPMENT OF OCULAR DOMINANCE COLUMNS

Geniculocortical Axons

Left-eye and right-eye inputs start out intermingled. The axons make and retract branches (Figure 11–10).

Relative Sizes of Ocular Dominance Columns

If both eyes are normal, each eye's inputs activate about equal numbers of cells. If the activity of one eye is reduced, the other eye will take over most of the territory.

Role of Activity

The N-methyl-D-aspartate (NMDA) type of glutamate receptor seems to play a pivotal role in the activity-dependent sorting out of connections. Spontaneous retinal activity before birth helps to initiate the sorting process. Visually elicited activity after birth is necessary to complete the process.

How do the patterns of ocular dominance columns develop? Are the geniculocortical axon terminals divided into left-eye and right-eye territories from the beginning? No. The initial geniculocortical projection to layer 4 is mixed (Figure 11–10).

Activity-Dependent Competition for Connections

The connections from the geniculate sort themselves out by making and breaking connections.

Most of this rearrangement takes place before birth, but the process continues for the first few years of life. Each eye will eventually control about 50% of layer 4. However, if one eye is not functioning properly during development, it will not get its share of cortical territory (Figure 11–11).

The more active axons compete more successfully for territory in layer 4, so most (but not all) of the cells in layer 4 will respond to the good eye and not the deprived eye, even if the ocular defect is eventually corrected.

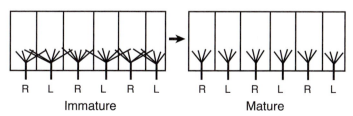

Figure 11–10
Geniculocortical axons initially branch widely in layer 4. The arbors are gradually remodeled to eliminate overlap between left-eye and right-eye zones.

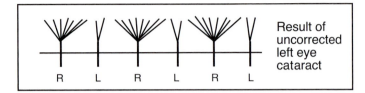

Result of uncorrected left eye cataract

R   L   R   L   R   L

Figure 11–11
If vision in one eye (the left eye in this example) is blocked during early postnatal life, the deprived eye's inputs will occupy as little as 20% rather than 50% of layer 4.

This dramatic effect happens only if there is a deficit during the critical period of development. Correlated patterns of activity are hypothesized to play a major role in the sorting-out process. This concept has been paraphrased: *axons that fire together, wire together.*

At birth, cortical layer 4 cells receive inputs from both sets of geniculate layers before the geniculocortical cells have completed their segregation. When an axon that conveys left-eye input to the cortical cell below becomes active, it helps change the state of the dendrite temporarily so that any other left-eye inputs become reinforced while axons that convey right-eye input become weakened. Eventually, the left-eye inputs take over in those cells. In the other 50% of layer 4 cells, right-eye inputs take over. If the left eye is deprived of vision at this time, the right-eye inputs can take over many of the cells that would normally be dominated by the left eye.

Spontaneous Waves

The sorting-out process begins before birth.

When these connections are beginning to sort out, there is no true visual input, but the retinas do have substantial *spontaneous wave activity*. Waves of activity are generated that sweep across the retina, producing waves of ganglion cell action potentials (Figure 11–12).

There is no correlation between the waves in the two eyes. Therefore, there will be correlations of activity for cells *within* each eye, but not *between* eyes.

How does this spontaneous activity help establish ocular dominance columns? A given axon conveying input, say, from the left eye, will fire in a pattern that is very similar to that of the axons relaying input from nearby regions of the left eye and that is less similar to the pattern of the axons relaying input from the right eye. Thus, left-eye axons will prefer to clump together with other left-eye axons and right-eye axons will prefer to terminate near other right-eye axons.

This pattern will be reinforced after birth, when visual input is available. If both eyes have normal input during development, then in layer 4 about half of the cells will be dominated by the right eye and the other half of the cells will be dominated by the left eye.

Mechanisms of Binocular Segregation

What events are triggered by activity that affects whether a connection is stabilized or retracted? In a basic feedback model, geniculocortical axons release glutamate, which in turn activates receptors that allow calcium to enter the dendrite; the calcium triggers release of a trophic factor that affects the structure of the geniculocortical synapse.

Glutamate Receptors

There is evidence that geniculocortical axons release glutamate as a transmitter. Molecules known as 2-(aminomethyl)phenylacetic acid (AMPA) receptors and N-methyl-D-aspartate (NMDA) receptors (two types of glutamate receptors) mediate the effect of firing on formation of ocular dominance columns.

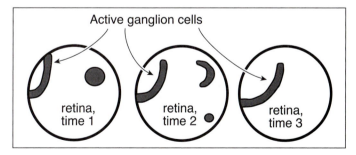

Figure 11–12
Waves of activity occur in retinal ganglion cells. The waves originate and travel in unpredictable patterns.

AMPA receptors allow sodium to flow into the dendrite and depolarize it. If several synapses are activated at the same time, each will be able to contribute to the depolarization that helps open NMDA channels. The resulting influx of calcium then sets off some as yet unknown process that stabilizes the synapses that just fired and also probably acts to destabilize the synapses that had not fired recently.

How would this mechanism explain the effects of monocular deprivation? The open eye would be more active than the closed eye and would trigger the NMDA-dependent mechanisms more successfully. Therefore, the open eye could take over more territory than normal, because its connections would be stabilized even in regions in which they were at first in the minority.

Changes in NMDA receptors are correlated with the critical period.

> Certain types of NMDA receptors may be required for activity-dependent organization of ocular dominance columns.

NMDA receptors are made up of different subunits that are expressed at different stages of development. Some subunits allow the channels to remain open for longer durations. NMDA-mediated excitatory postsynaptic currents (EPSCs) in layer 4 neurons of the visual cortex last longer in young rats than in adult rats, and the durations of the EPSCs become progressively shorter, in parallel with the developmental reduction in synaptic plasticity. Also, NMDA receptor density in cortex is greater in early life than in later life, and the decrease in receptors may limit plasticity.

Retrograde Messengers

> The NMDA model suggests that activated dendrites release a substance that helps to sustain inputs with appropriate activity.

For example, axons may compete for brain-derived neurotrophic factor (BDNF) or some other substance. If one eye is deprived, then those axons do not get enough BDNF and they shrink. In support of this idea, BDNF mRNA is found in the cortex during the critical period. Also, the receptor to which BDNF binds (trkB) is present.

If axons are competing for a limited amount of BDNF, then supplying excess factor should allow all the axons to retain their connections. This idea has been tested by infusing BDNF into the cortex of kittens during the period within which segregation of columns normally takes place. As predicted, an oversupply of BDNF allows axons to stay mixed together, and columns do not appear. If axons are competing for a limited amount of BDNF, then reducing the levels of BDNF in the cortex should result in reduced axon growth. As predicted, there is a lower overall branching of axons in the affected region.

Orientation Columns

Are other aspects of cortical organization influenced by activity during development? The role of activity has been examined in the development of orientation columns.

> Anatomical studies show that in the mature cortex, cells in a given orientation column have connections with cells in other columns with a similar orientation preference.

Patchy zones of connections develop gradually (Figure 11–13).

Surprisingly, retinal activity is not required for this development. However, the cortex and lateral geniculate also have the ability to fire spontaneous bursts. If this intrinsic activity is blocked, the clusters do not form. Therefore the cortex (or the geniculocortical complex) is also a potential source of spontaneous activity that may help to shape the connections of the developing cortex.

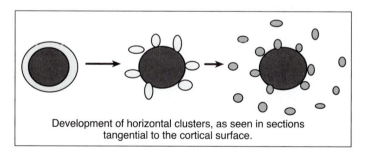

Development of horizontal clusters, as seen in sections tangential to the cortical surface.

Figure 11–13
Anatomical methods show that a given patch of cortex (black areas) is initially connected to a uniform "halo" of cells. Over time, some connections are lost and others develop, leaving connections primarily between patches of cells with similar orientation preferences.

BEYOND THE STRIATE CORTEX

What happens to the information processed in the striate cortex? It is distributed directly or indirectly to many locations in the brain, including dozens of regions of the cortex. At least 30 regions of the cortex play a role in visual perception or visually guided movement. The many visual areas in the cortex have been roughly divided into two categories.

> Some areas are mostly involved in determining *what* an object is, and other areas are mostly involved in determining *where* an object is.

The What Stream

> The *what stream* is an assemblage of areas, particularly in the temporal cortex, that contain cells that are particularly sensitive to details of shape and form.

For example, some areas contain cells that respond to complex distributions of patterns. As in the striate cortex, there seems to be a columnar arrangement, so that similar shapes activate the cells in a given column. An even higher level of specificity is found in the fusiform gyrus in humans, in which cells are particularly active in response to faces. In comparable areas in the monkey, individual cells can be found that respond best to faces of monkeys and humans. Damage to different parts of the temporal *what* stream can produce *agnosia,* a syndrome in which a person may be able to see an object but yet be unable to identify it by sight; such a person might be able to identify a pencil by touching it but not by looking at it. Another type of lesion can produce *prosopagnosia,* a loss of ability to recognize people, even one's self, by sight. In addition, the perception of color seems to be mediated by cells in the ventral stream. Damage to some of these areas can lead to loss of ability to see colors: the world appears to be black, white, and gray.

The Where Stream

> The *where stream* is an assemblage of areas in the occipitoparietal region. Cells in these regions are particularly sensitive to perception of the location and movement of objects, including one's own movements.

In some parts of the *where* stream, cells show a strong preference for moving stimuli rather than stationary stimuli. Some of the preferences can be quite specific, such as for cells that respond best to spiral movements. Still farther along in the pathway are cells that respond best when an object is moving toward the body, cells that respond preferentially to an object that is within arm's reach, and so forth. Lesions in these areas can lead to difficulties in perceiving movement. For example, after such a lesion, a person might have problems in estimating how fast an oncoming car is traveling: it might seem to be far away and then suddenly to be close at hand. Other lesions can interfere with the ability to pre-position one's hand correctly when picking up an object. A person with this sort of lesion might have no difficulty recognizing a pencil, but would be unable to position his or her hand appropriately when trying to remove the pencil from a table top.

Although this division of the higher visual areas into *what* and *where* streams has a real core of truth to it, the division is by no means absolute. There are interconnections between regions of the two streams, and, in ways not yet understood, we must be able to integrate the two sorts of information so that we can make sense of a diverse visual scene in which some objects may be moving while others are stationary. This need for integration has been termed the *binding problem*. Some researchers hypothesize that groups of cells in different visual areas fire more synchronously when they are activated by the same object than by different objects. The resolution to this puzzle awaits future electrophysiological and imaging studies in animals and humans.

Attention

Another area of active study is that of attention. Evidence is accumulating to show that shifting attention from one object to another can modulate the responses of cells in many parts of the brain. How this shift is initiated and controlled is still an unsolved question.

· C H A P T E R · 1 2 ·

THE NEUROBIOLOGY OF MEMORY

·

Kathleen M. K. Boje

Types of Memory: A Cognitive Overview

The Importance of Various Neural Systems in Learning and Memory

The Scientific Debate on the Basis of Memory Formation:
  Synaptic versus Neurochemical Signal-Transduction Mechanisms

Molecular Mechanisms for the Establishment of Long-Term Memory

Neurotransmitter Modulation of Memory Processes

Effects of Aging and Neurological Pathologies on Learning and Memory

Overview

·   ·   ·   ·   ·   ·   ·   ·   ·   ·   ·   ·

Learning is the ability to acquire new information, whereas *memory* is the ability to retain and recall that information over time.

As such, learning and memory processes can be studied and understood from a variety of different perspectives—cognitive psychology, educational psychology, cognitive neuroscience, functional neuroimaging, and neurobiology at the systemic, cellular, and molecular levels. The objective of this chapter is to introduce a neurobiological overview of the mechanisms of memory.

TYPES OF MEMORY: A COGNITIVE OVERVIEW

Memory is often categorized based on the length of time that information is retained. Memory is classified as short-term, working, or long-term memory.

1. *Short-term memory* involves the retention or awareness of information for a brief moment.
2. *Working memory* involves the retention of information for a period of time sufficient for a cognitive process to occur. The information is then forgotten.
3. *Long-term memory* involves the retention of information that did not occur recently. It can be classified into declarative (facts) or nondeclarative (skills, habits, and procedures).

Short-term memory is a memory of an event that just occurred. A limited amount of information is retained only briefly, unless there is a deliberate effort to rehearse and retain it. Working memory, a contemporary alternative to short-term memory, refers to a process(es) in which information is temporarily stored while it is presently being used. Long-term memory is a recollection of an event that is not currently held in attention. Recall of long-term memories may require some effort ("jogging one's memory").

Working Memory

The brain processes much information as daily activities are carried out. This information is usually retained in working memory, utilized, then forgotten. For example, working memory permits you to perform simple mathematical calculations in your head or remember a phone number long enough to dial it. It also permits you to analyze and creatively interpret data without creating a permanent memory. Information stored in working memory is akin to a brief scribble on a disposable Post-it note.

Long-Term Memory:
Declarative (Explicit) versus Nondeclarative (Implicit)

Long-term memory can be subclassified into declarative (explicit) or non-declarative (implicit) memory.

> Explicit or *declarative memory* encompasses the conscious, willful retrieval of information that can be verbalized.

It often involves information about people, places, or things, such as the remembrance of a favorite teacher. Explicit memory may be further subdivided into episodic and semantic memory. Episodic memory involves conscious retrieval of memories that constitute our personal life, such as meeting a friend for the first time. Semantic memory is knowledge that permits us to function in life without the necessity for deliberate, conscious recollection. Examples of semantic memory involve activities such as telling time, making change for a $20 bill, or preparing a pizza.

Alternatively, the implicit (nondeclarative) form of long-term memory does not depend on a conscious effort.

> *Nondeclarative memory* often involves an unintentional remembering of skills and habits.

Procedural memory, or remembering how to do a procedure, is another type of implicit memory. Examples of implicit memory involve activities such as riding a bicycle or walking.

Cognitive Storage and Organization of Memories

Information can be stored in long-term memory deliberately, by individual choice; this is generally accomplished by rehearsing and reinforcing the information. However, information may often be stored in long-term memory without a deliberate conscious decision. The hippocampus plays a role in this. Information is most likely to be retained long-term when the information has emotional significance and/or when the information is related to an existing knowledge base.

The brain does not retain random bits of information, but rather, organizes information and links it to what is already learned and retained in a process called *elaborative encoding*. For example, the name of a person just met is readily forgotten if the only information link is the person's face. However, as more is learned about the person, the person's name becomes linked to informative details and impressions. The stronger the web of information about the person, the better the encoding process linking the person's name to the information, and, hence, the greater probability the person's name will be recalled.

THE IMPORTANCE OF VARIOUS NEURAL SYSTEMS IN LEARNING AND MEMORY

Declarative and nondeclarative memories invoke the participation of different neural systems. Implicit processes, involving motor skills, habits, or procedures, activate neuronal sensory and motor systems (e.g., the brainstem, cerebellum, and cortex). Interestingly, the storage of these types of memories is generally conserved among lower mammals and humans. Explicit processes activate the hippocampus and regions of the temporal cerebral cortex, basal forebrain, and thalamus. Because explicit (declarative) memory information can often be verbalized, these types of memories are generally stored in the phylogenetically newer neuronal connections involving the thalamus, cortical temporal lobes, and hippocampus.

Clinical and experimental data indicate that

> the formation of long-term memories is critically dependent on interactions among the medial temporal lobe, the hippocampal system (and associated cortex), and the neocortex.

Serious memory impairments occur after hippocampal damage or injury to the neuronal connections between the hippocampus and the neocortex.

The Role of the Hippocampus

The hippocampus is critical in the formation of explicit memories.

> The hippocampus is intimately involved in the conversion of short-term memories into long-term memories, a process known as *consolidation.*

Consolidation occurs over a protracted period of time (days to years). One theory proposes that consolidation involves hippocampal coordination of multiple stimuli and activation to strengthen the association of information previously stored in the neocortex. Hence long-term memories are stored and recalled from the neocortex, but this can occur only after the hippocampus has "conditioned" the neocortex for memory storage.

The Case of H.M. Clinical case studies of people who incurred permanent hippocampal injury have revealed the role of the hippocampus in the consolidation process. From these cases, it is inferred that damage to the hippocampus does not impair the ability to recall old memories, but does impair the ability to form new memories.

The classic example illustrating the importance of the hippocampus in the process of learning and memory is the story of H.M., a Connecticut factory worker. H.M. suffered from severe, intractable, drug-resistant epilepsy. Subsequent surgical removal of the hippocampus and several neighboring structures (including the amygdala) effectively reduced the frequency and severity of H.M.'s seizures, but, unfortunately, also impaired his learning and memory processes. H.M. was afflicted with moderate retrograde amnesia (loss of memory for events occurring shortly prior to brain damage) and severe anterograde amnesia (loss of memory for events occurring after brain damage). He retained the memories of events preceding the surgery, and did have an intact short-term memory, but could not consolidate the short-term memories into permanent storage. In other words, H.M. had fleeting short-term memories, but could not form long-term memories. For example, H.M. could converse with the hospital staff, but could not remember them even though he saw them every day.

Although H.M. was unable to learn and retain new information, he was able to acquire motor skills without much difficulty. For example, he could learn the mechanical skills required to play golf, although he could not remember ever learning those skills. In summary, the loss of the hippocampus left H.M. with an impaired declarative memory—he was unable to recall and verbally describe a memory; however, his procedural memory (the ability to learn and retain motor skills) was left intact.

THE SCIENTIFIC DEBATE ON THE BASIS OF MEMORY FORMATION: SYNAPTIC VERSUS NEUROCHEMICAL SIGNAL-TRANSDUCTION MECHANISMS

A precise understanding of the mechanisms underlying the neurobiology of memory storage remains elusive and is the focus of intense research, controversy, and passion. There is general agreement that information stored into memory requires changes in neuronal physiology. The various competing hypotheses share a common belief that the cellular basis of memory is derived from persistent changes among neurons involved in the neuronal networks of information storage. However, the precise mechanisms of these persistent changes—alterations of the functional synapse versus alterations in neuronal signal-transduction mechanisms—are the subject of intense debate.

Two hypotheses describe the neuronal creation and storage of memories: a synaptically-based mechanism and a neurochemical signal-transduction-based mechanism.

Central to the synaptic hypothesis is the concept that memory storage results from alterations in the effectiveness of individual synapses between neurons, which occur through the electrophysiological phenomena of long-term potentiation (LTP) and long-term depression (LTD). The neurochemical signal-transduction hypothesis maintains that memories are formed and stored through depolarization-triggered alterations in molecular events leading to and from elevations in cytosolic calcium. Table 12–1 presents an overview of and Figure 12–1 illustrates several important differences between the two hypotheses of memory creation and storage.

Table 12–1   OVERVIEW OF THE CURRENT HYPOTHESES OF MEMORY FORMATION: THE SYNAPTIC BASIS OF MEMORY VERSUS THE NEUROCHEMICAL BASIS OF MEMORY

The Synaptic Hypothesis
- Depolarization evokes changes in the effectiveness of individual synapses between neurons.
- Long-term potentiation (LTP) and long-term depression (LTD) are electrophysiological phenomena that represent a mechanism altering the "strength" or synaptic activity that a synapse exerts on its postsynaptic cell.
- LTP or LTD evokes Ca^{2+} influx via excitatory glutamate receptors (predominantly N-methyl-D-aspartate and α-amino-3-hydroxy-5-methyl-4-isoxazolepropionic acid subtypes) to initiate a series of downstream events resulting in persistent synaptic modifications for information storage.
- Synaptic electrophysiological activities (manifested by LTP or LTD) persist for the duration of the memory.

The Neurochemical Hypothesis
- Neuronal depolarization (via activation of G-protein-coupled receptors, ligand-gated ion channels, or voltage-gated ion channels) elicits release of intracellular calcium from internal calcium pools.
- Elevated intracellular calcium promotes the autophosphorylation of various kinases, for example, protein kinase C and calcium/calmodulin-dependent kinase (CaMKII) and activation of calexcitin, a calcium-binding protein.
- These calcium-dependent kinases (calexcitin, protein kinase C, and CaMKII) act to inhibit synaptic potassium channels, thereby causing the neuronal membrane to become readily susceptible to further depolarization events.

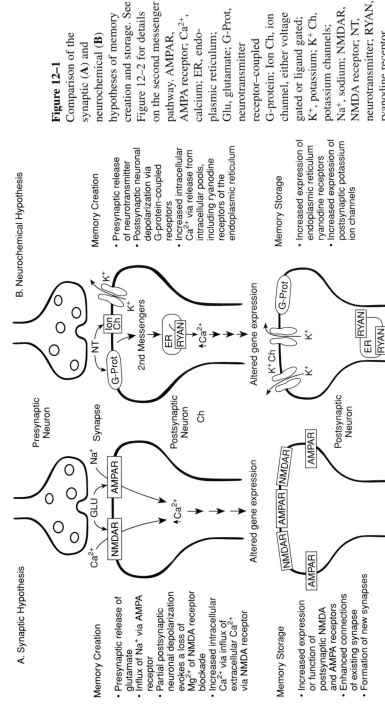

A. Synaptic Hypothesis

B. Neurochemical Hypothesis

Memory Creation

- Presynaptic release of glutamate
- Influx of Na^+ via AMPA receptor
- Partial postsynaptic neuronal depolarization evokes a loss of Mg^{2+} of NMDA receptor blockade
- Increased intracellular Ca^{2+} via influx of extracellular Ca^{2+} via NMDA receptor

Memory Storage

- Increased expression or function of postsynaptic NMDA and AMPA receptors
- Enhanced connections of existing synapse
- Formation of new synapses

Memory Creation

- Presynaptic release of neurotransmitter
- Postsynaptic neuronal depolarization via G-protein-coupled receptors
- Increased intracellular Ca^{2+} via release from intracellular pools, including ryanodine receptors of the endoplasmic reticulum

Memory Storage

- Increased expression of endoplasmic reticulum ryanodine receptors
- Increased expression of postsynaptic potassium ion channels

Figure 12–1

Comparison of the synaptic (**A**) and neurochemical (**B**) hypotheses of memory creation and storage. See Figure 12–2 for details on the second messenger pathway. AMPAR, AMPA receptor; Ca^{2+}, calcium; ER, endoplasmic reticulum; Glu, glutamate; G-Prot, neurotransmitter receptor–coupled G-protein; Ion Ch, ion channel, either voltage gated or ligand gated; K^+, potassium; K^+ Ch, potassium channels; Na^+, sodium; NMDAR, NMDA receptor; NT, neurotransmitter; RYAN, ryanodine receptor.

234

A Synaptic Mechanism of Memory

> The synaptic hypothesis of memory induction and storage proposes that the synapse is the critical site for memory.

Use-dependent changes occur via repeated electrical depolarization and serve to modify the synapse in a manner conducive for mechanisms of memory. The electrophysiological phenomena of long-term potentiation and long-term depression are critically implicated in a synaptic mechanism of memory.

What Is Long-Term Potentiation and Long-Term Depression?   Long-term potentiation and long-term depression are electrophysiological phenomena that represent a mechanism for synaptic activity associated with processes of learning and memory.

> *Long-term potentiation* (LTP) and *long-term depression* (LTD) represent the "strength" or effects that a synapse has on its postsynaptic cell: LTP represents a stronger synaptic effect and LTD represents a weaker synaptic effect.

Under certain conditions of synaptic activation, the synaptic strength can be adjusted upward (LTP) or downward (LTD), and the synapse will retain that strength until new conditions are presented. The term *synaptic plasticity* refers to changes in the strength of synapses.

In simplistic terms, LTP describes a long-lasting (hours in vitro; days in vivo) enhancement of synaptic neurotransmission following rapid, high-frequency electrical presynaptic stimulation. LTP occurs when a synapse is rapidly and repetitively stimulated, concurrently with depolarization of neighboring synapses impinging on the same neuron. LTD occurs when the synapse is activated infrequently without activation of neighboring synapses. Both LTP and LTD are electrophysiological processes occurring at synapses that involve persistent changes in synaptic strength following persistent electrical neurotransmission across synapses.

How Is LTP/LTD Induced?

> LTP occurs in neuronal pathways when electrical tetanic stimulation of presynaptic neuronal inputs causes a lasting increase in the efficacy of synaptic neurotransmission, as measured in the postsynaptic neuron.

Stated another way, LTP is a generalized, prolonged enhancement of excitatory postsynaptic potentials (EPSPs), which represent the electrical charges in the postsynaptic neuronal membrane that contribute to the generation of an action potential.

The in vitro expression of LTP was first described in the rabbit hippocampus. Although LTP can occur in various regions of the brain (e.g., hippocampus and cerebral cortex), hippocampal LTP is well studied in vitro, in part because of the easy identification and access of the hippocampal neurocircuitry. LTP is induced by electrical stimulation of a neuron with a brief, rapid train of stimuli (e.g., 100 synaptic excitations over a 1-sec time interval), after which the neuron is said to be in a potentiated state. Following LTP, the neuron is highly responsive to new stimuli for a very long period of time.

LTD, in contrast, represents a weakening of synaptic strength. It is induced by low-frequency (1-Hz) electrical stimuli (e.g., one synaptic excitation per second over a 1-min interval). LTD is thought to reverse persistent LTP.

The Attractiveness of LTP as a Neurobiological Model of Learning and Memory   LTP represents an electrophysiological model of learning and memory in that a variety of stimulatory changes occur that either facilitate or decrease the activity of neuronal synapses. LTP has several distinguishing characteristics that make it an attractive neurobiological model of learning and memory.

> LTP shows the characteristics of *cooperativity* and *associativity.*

Cooperativity describes the situation in which simultaneous stimulation of a neuron by two or more neighboring axons will produce LTP in the postsynaptic neuron. Associativity occurs when a postsynaptic neuron receives a weak stimulating input concurrent with a strong stimulating input. Thereafter, the postsynaptic neuron will later respond to the weak input without the necessity of having the strong input.

Cellular Mechanisms of LTP: Involvement of Glutamate Receptors   Although the precise cellular mechanisms underlying the induction of LTP remain a focus of research, it is clear that mechanisms based on simple alterations in neurotransmitter release or changes in dendritic spine resistances do not singularly account for LTP. The important feature of the synaptic hypothesis is that Ca^{2+} influx via glutamate receptors serves as a signal-transduction mechanism that is vitally important for induction of LTP (see Figure 12–1A). These processes initiate persistent synaptic modifications during a consolidation process.

Though not fully understood, the induction and maintenance of LTP require both presynaptic and postsynaptic events at excitatory glutaminergic synapses.

> Induction of LTP requires a series of coordinated events involving intense neuronal depolarization, enhanced glutamate release from presynaptic vesicles, and activation of specific subsets of postsynaptic glutamate receptors.

This is followed by intracellular increases in neuronal calcium levels, enhanced calcium/calmodulin-dependent kinase II function, activation-specific tyrosine kinases, and other as yet unknown neurochemical cascades (Figure 12–2).

Early research focused heavily on the involvement of a specific postsynaptic glutamate receptor subtype, the N-methyl-D-aspartate (NMDA) receptors.

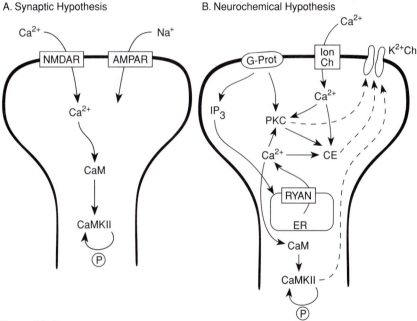

Figure 12–2
Simplified illustration of the second messenger pathways involved in the synaptic (**A**) and neurochemical (**B**) hypotheses of memory creation. Solid arrows represent stimulating events; dashed arrows represent inhibitory events. AMPAR, AMPA receptor; Ca^{2+}, calcium; CaM, calmodulin; CaMKII, calcium/calmodulin-dependent kinase; CE, calexcitin; ER, endoplasmic reticulum; G-Prot, neurotransmitter receptor-coupled G-protein; Ion Ch, ion channel, either voltage gated or ligand gated; IP_3, inositol triphosphate; K^+, potassium; NMDAR, NMDA receptor; P, phosphorylation process; PKC, protein kinase C.

However, recent research implicates the involvement of another postsynaptic glutamate receptor subtype, the α-amino-3-hydroxy-5-methyl-4-isoxazolepropionic acid (AMPA) receptor. Several reports provide a fascinating picture of a concerted role for AMPA and NMDA during LTP (or LTD)-induced modulation of synaptic strength.

AMPA and NMDA receptors are ideally suited for induction of LTP (of LTD) because these receptors are localized postsynaptically on neurons known to undergo LTP (LTD).

> *AMPA receptors* are ligand-gated cationic (predominately sodium) channels that are responsible for fast excitatory neurotransmission.

AMPA receptors respond quickly to synaptically released glutamate following depolarization of the presynaptic neuron. In contrast,

> *NMDA receptors* are ligand-gated cationic channels, with a large calcium conductance, that are responsible for slower and prolonged neurotransmission.

Activation of excitatory NMDA receptors requires the binding of two neurotransmitters, glutamate and glycine, and partial depolarization (to remove the magnesium blockade of the ion channel). AMPA-mediated influx of sodium ions elicits a partial depolarization of the postsynaptic neuron, thereby relieving the voltage-gated magnesium block of the NMDA receptor. Calcium and sodium currents then flux through the NMDA receptors for relatively prolonged periods of time (e.g., a few hundreds of milliseconds).

Elegant research studies suggest that it is the dynamic, plastic regulation of postsynaptic AMPA and NMDA receptors that governs the strength of the synaptic connection following LTP (or LTD) induction. After induction of LTP, there is an enhanced recruitment of postsynaptic AMPA receptors and an enhanced recruitment (or altered subunit composition) of NMDA receptors. Moreover, LTP-induced kinase activation may promote receptor subunit phosphorylation, which assists in receptor trafficking to the postsynaptic membrane and enhancement of channel ion conductance. These events have the subsequent effect of increased synaptic efficacy. Conversely, after LTD, fewer AMPA receptors were localized to the postsynaptic membrane.

Relationship Between LTP and Animal Learning and Memory Tasks
Hippocampal LTP/LTD is widely studied, in part because of the simplicity of the

neuronal circuitry (relative to other brain regions) and the accrued evidence linking hippocampal function and short-term memory in humans and animals. Several different strategies have been used to determine whether LTP serves as a mechanism for memory. The Morris water maze test is frequently used as a learning and memory paradigm for spatial memory in rodents. However, contrasting relationships between LTP and rodent performance in the Morris water maze test have been shown. LTP has been manipulated through the use of conventional drugs (or antisense molecules). Pharmacological inhibition of hippocampal NMDA receptors blocked induction of LTP and produced impaired performance in the water maze test. In addition, transgenic NMDA mice (knockout of the $\epsilon1$ or NR2A subunit or deletion of the NMDAR1 subunit in the hippocampal CA1 region) exhibited impaired hippocampal LTP and impaired performance in the Morris water maze test. In other studies, the mechanism for LTP induction was saturated in vivo to determine if additional learning was possible. Animals subsequently were impaired in learning new tasks. Collectively, these studies ostensibly provide a link between LTP and spatial memory tasks.

However, as a description of the processes of memory, LTP is too simplistic. Pretraining rodents in one Morris water maze followed by pharmacological blockade of NMDA receptors did not impair spatial learning in a different water maze configuration, yet impaired electrophysiological expression of LTP was observed. These unexpected findings prompted a rethinking of the role of NMDA receptors in the Morris water maze learning and memory paradigm. In addition, equivocal impairment of rodent learning and memory tasks was observed following saturation of LTP. Other studies utilizing transgenic mice (AMPA knockouts or NMDA overexpression of the NR2D subunit) revealed inconsistencies in the relationship between LTP and spatial memory. In particular, severe impairments in LTP were observed in the various transgenic mice, yet performance in the Morris water maze was essentially normal. In a different experimental paradigm, antisense molecules specific for presynaptic potassium channels were injected into rodent hippocampus. The antisense treatment successfully elicited a reduced expression of the channel and eliminated LTP, yet did not alter rodent performance in the Morris water maze.

The best available evidence to date does not clearly correlate LTP with processes of learning and memory.

One complicating factor is an increasing awareness among researchers that LTP may not be a homogeneous phenomenon, but in fact may be heterogeneous. Researchers are beginning to distinguish the existence of LTP in different temporal forms: early LTP, which begins immediately after a single, high-frequency electrical stimulus train, and late LTP, which is manifest a few hours after three or four serially spaced, high-frequency stimulus trains and persists for 8 or more hours thereafter.

> *Early LTP* is dependent on short-term second messenger alterations (e.g., kinase activity), whereas *late LTP* is dependent on de novo gene transcription and protein synthesis.

Another critically important obstacle in correlating LTP with learning and memory is that LTP is particularly difficult to observe in the intact animal *during* a learning and memory task. Attempts to observe LTP is complicated by the fact that we do not know which synapses to monitor for LTP, largely because searching for LTP among an array of synapses is akin to searching for a needle in a haystack. Moreover, it becomes even more challenging to observe LTP after long-term storage of the memory in the intact animal, again because of the difficulty in localizing particular synapses for electrophysiological monitoring.

Neurochemical Signal-Transduction-Based Mechanism of Memory

Not all scientists agree that LTP is an adequate mechanism to describe learning and memory. Some argue that LTP is an overly simplistic representation of a complicated neurobiological mechanism. Others assert that although LTP may occur, it is neither necessary nor sufficient for memory. Hence an alternative neurochemical hypothesis may provide a basis for understanding the molecular basis of memory.

The Critical Role of Intracellular Calcium

> Central to the neurochemical signal-transduction process is the hypothesis that phasic changes in intracellular calcium will elicit various downstream, long-lasting cellular events.

Neuronal depolarization occurs via a variety of mechanisms: activation of G-protein-coupled receptors, ligand-gated ion channels, or voltage-gated ion channels. Subsequent increases in intracellular calcium occur predominantly by release of calcium from intracellular organelles (see Figure 12–1B). Although influx of calcium through ion channels can and does occur, this source of increased intracellular calcium is relatively smaller in magnitude and duration than release via intracellular pools.

Temporal Phases of Intracellular Calcium Signaling Elevated intracellular calcium triggers a variety of neurochemical signal-transduction cascades (see Figure 12–2). These cascades occur over a period of milliseconds to days, with the ultimate effect of promoting neuronal excitability and synaptic efficacy.

During the initial depolarization phase, intracellular calcium is elevated, either by extracellular calcium influx via ion channels or by receptor–G-protein-coupled increases in phosphoinositol and subsequent endoplasmic release of intracellular calcium. Over the next milliseconds to seconds, increased intracellular calcium promotes the autophosphorylation of various kinases, such as protein kinase C and calcium/calmodulin-dependent kinase (CaMKII), thereby causing the activity of these kinases to become independent of calcium signaling.

In the next time frame (seconds to minutes), increased intracellular calcium and protein kinase C activity act in concert to activate calexcitin, a calcium-binding protein. Calexcitin controls intracellular calcium by two separate mechanisms. First, it amplifies calcium signaling through promotion of intracellular calcium release by endoplasmic reticulum ryanodine receptors. Following a period of elevated intracellular calcium, calexcitin activates endoplasmic reticulum calcium-ATPase to resequester intracellular calcium back in the endoplasmic reticulum. Second, calexcitin translocates to the membrane, whereupon calexcitin, protein kinase C, and CaMKII act to inhibit synaptic potassium channels. Inhibition of these channels has a net effect of rendering the neuronal membrane more excitable by further depolarization events.

Over the course of minutes to hours, intracellular calcium and calexcitin act indirectly on transcriptional factors to enhance gene transcription and subsequent protein synthesis. Enhanced expression of ryanodine receptors at the endoplasmic reticulum and inhibition of potassium channels at the synapse serve to maintain enhanced neuronal susceptibility to depolarization. A variety of different proteins are synthesized, including proteins related to axonal transport and to structural remodeling of the neuron and synapse.

MOLECULAR MECHANISMS FOR THE ESTABLISHMENT OF LONG-TERM MEMORY

Memories are stored for long periods of time. The two hypotheses of memory, LTP versus neurochemical signal transduction, differ in describing how and where memories are formed and stored. The LTP hypothesis proposes that persistent electrophysiological changes in activated synapses underlie the retention of information. Thus, it is believed that prolonged maintenance and sustained duration of LTP are required for memory storage. To some extent, this may also encompass morphological changes in synaptic structure and/or numbers. The neurochemical signal-transduction hypothesis maintains that alterations in neurobiochemistry and molecular neurobiology, as regulated by differential intracellular calcium signaling, are the basis of memory storage. Regardless of which hypothesis is advocated, the following is certain:

the creation and maintenance (i.e., *memory consolidation*) of permanent memories involve a dynamic process involving electrical processes, neurochemical processes, or both to prime neurons for memory consolidation.

Involvement of Increased Intracellular Calcium

During the information acquisition phase, both hypotheses involve alterations in the levels of intracellular calcium. However, the mechanisms that precede the alterations are, for each hypothesis, differently invoked.

The LTP hypothesis invokes active participation of postsynaptic glutamate receptors (the fast-acting AMPA and protracted contribution of the NMDA receptor) during presynaptic electrical depolarization.

Intracellular calcium rises as a result of the influx of calcium via the NMDA receptor.

The neurochemical signal-transduction hypothesis invokes neuronal depolarization through a variety of receptor-mediated and cation channels.

The subsequent neuronal depolarization elicits release of calcium from two sources: either influx of calcium through cationic channels or release of calcium from intracellular pools found in various organelles, such as the endoplasmic reticulum, sarcoplasmic reticulum, and mitochondria. Increased intracellular calcium elicits the activation of a variety of proteins involved in signal transduction.

Involvement of Signal-Transduction Events

Elevation of postsynaptic intracellular calcium levels is not sufficient for the induction and maintenance of long-term memory. Activation of various phosphatases and kinases is important.

Phosphatase activation occurs under conditions of low intracellular calcium levels, as might occur during LTD. Conversely, kinase activation [e.g., calcium/

calmodulin-dependent protein kinase II (CaMKII), protein kinases A and C] occurs with high intracellular calcium levels, as would occur during LTP. Once activated, CaMKII undergoes autophosphorylation, thereby becoming independent of intracellular calcium levels. CaMKII then phosphorylates a variety of proteins, including glutamate receptors, cyclic adenylyl monophosphate responsive element-binding protein (CREB), and neurofilaments. Protein kinase C (PKC) stimulates adenylyl cyclase with the subsequent formation of cyclic adenylyl monophosphate (cAMP). cAMP is implicated in altering gene expression (see below).

Involvement of Gene Expression and Protein Synthesis

Considerable research has been conducted on the mechanisms of conversion of short-term memories into long-term memories.

> Research on both forms of learning, implicit and explicit, suggests that gene-mediated events result in new protein synthesis, which is vital for conversion of short-term to long-term memories.

For example, a generalized increase in soluble neuronal proteins was observed during and in the early hours following a learning task, followed by an increase in membrane-bound proteins in later stages, 4–8 hours after the learning experience. Formation of short-term memories and recall of established long-term memories were not altered by application of nonspecific mRNA and protein synthesis inhibitors, whereas these pharmacological interventions did disrupt the formation of new, long-term memories. Although the precise identities of specific induced proteins are presently unknown, it is possible that these proteins may represent regulatory proteins involved in the remodeling of neuronal connections and/or synaptically localized receptors and ion channels.

At the molecular level, several cascades are involved in altering gene expression. CREB is a nuclear transcription factor that, once activated, regulates gene expression. It is phosphorylated as a result of increased cAMP and subsequent protein kinase A (PKA) activity or by CaMKII.

Enhanced gene expression and protein synthesis are common themes of the two different models of memory storage. The LTP synaptic model suggests that alterations in the synapses, either by altered expression of NMDA and AMPA receptors, increased expression of new synapses, and/or new synaptic connections, underlie memory storage (see Figure 12–1A). The neurochemical signal-transduction model suggests that increased expression of intracellular calcium-releasing ryanodine receptors and voltage-dependent potassium channels forms the molecular basis of long-term memory (see Figure 12–1B).

Current Hypotheses on the "Molecular Switches" that Maintain Memories

Several biochemical cascades may serve as molecular switches to "turn on" the formation and retention of a memory. These biochemical cascades serve as positive feedback loops to initiate and maintain stable memories. Several molecular mechanisms have been proposed (Figure 12–3):

> a second messenger switch, a kinase switch, a transcriptional switch, a transitional switch, and a structural unit switch composed of protein subunits at the pre- and postsynaptic membrane.

All of these molecular mechanisms can be activated by a strong stimulus and can be self-sustaining after the initial stimulus via a positive feedforward loop. Hence these various candidate mechanisms are attractive explanations for a molecular basis of memory.

Two of the hypothesized molecular switches involve signal-transduction events (see Figure 12–3A). One second messenger mechanism involves the

A. Signal Transduction

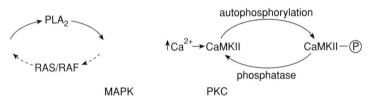

MAPK   PKC

B. Altered Gene Expression

CREB → → → ↑ Gene expression and protein synthesis

"dormant" mRNA $\overrightarrow{CPEB}$ polyadenylated mRNA → → ↑ protein synthesis

Figure 12–3
Hypothesized molecular "switches" that may maintain memories. (**A**) Signal transduction; (**B**) altered gene expression. Solid arrows represent stimulating events; dashed arrows represent positive feedforward events. Ca^{2+}, calcium; CaMKII, calcium/calmodulin-dependent kinase; CPEB, cytoplasmic polyadenylation element-binding protein; CREB, cAMP-responsive element-binding protein; MAPK, mitogen-activated protein kinase; PKC, protein kinase C; PLA_2, phospholipase A_2.

mitogen-activated protein kinases (MAPK) and activation of protein kinase C (via phospholipase A_2). Once activated, protein kinase C can feedforward to activate MAPK through Ras/Raf. The other second messenger mechanism involves a kinase switch. In this situation, CaMKII will autophosphorylate several of its subunits in the presence of elevated intracellular calcium. Following autophosphorylation, CaMKII activity becomes independent of calcium levels. If one CaMKII subunit undergoes dephosphorylation by a phosphatase, the other phosphorylated CaMKII subunits can rephosphorylate the subunit, thereby ensuring that the kinase is continually activated.

Two other hypothesized molecular switches involve alterations in gene expression. One mechanism involves a transcriptional switch (see Figure 12–3B). The transcription factor, CREB, is involved in signal-transduction events that regulate gene expression. Activation of CREB leads to enhanced gene expression of products that augment CREB and other transcription factors. Hence, this feedforward mechanism involving a transcriptional "turning on" of gene expression may provide yet another basis for stable memories. The other molecular switch involves a translational mechanism. Translationally dormant mRNA residing in proximity to a synapse is polyadenylated by cytoplasmic polyadenylation element-binding (CPEB) protein. CPEB is likely activated by second messengers arising from synaptic activity. One candidate protein that arises from this mechanism is CaMKII.

The last two mechanisms of molecular memory storage involve alterations or stabilization in the structural organization of the synapse. The subunits resident in the presynaptic and postsynaptic membranes may be stabilized by a steady-state replacement of subunits during protein turnover. Alternatively, a very stable protein may insert into the organization of the synapse, thereby stabilizing the synapse subunits and conferring protection from protein degradation.

NEUROTRANSMITTER MODULATION OF MEMORY PROCESSES

> Synaptic neurotransmitters influence memory processes, either positively or negatively.

Glutamate is a neurotransmitter in the forefront, primarily because of its prominent excitatory role within the hippocampal and cortical regions, as previously discussed. Acetylcholinergic neurons project from the nucleus basalis to the cortex and may augment the actions of glutamate. Atropine, a muscarinic acetylcholine receptor antagonist, causes amnesia in humans. Release of the inhibitory neurotransmitter γ-aminobutyric acid (GABA) impairs memory, possibly by interfering with neuronal excitation and/or attenuating the activity of the cholinergic projections to the cortex. Biogenic amines, such as norepinephrine, dopamine, or serotonin, may influence memory formation and retention. Lastly, various neuropeptides and trophic proteins may also modulate memory through activation of receptors and signal-transduction pathways in the neural networks involved in memory.

EFFECTS OF AGING AND NEUROLOGICAL PATHOLOGIES ON LEARNING AND MEMORY

A variety of disease conditions can alter learning and memory processes.

Some of these conditions arise from genetics, life-styles (i.e., nutritional deficiencies and alcoholism), or neurodegenerative diseases. Brief overviews of various medical conditions involving disturbances in memory processes follow.

Aging

Contrary to popular perception, aging does not impair the processes of learning and memory.

Diseases such as high blood pressure, thyroid dysfunction, depression or anxiety disorder, or other conditions such as chronic stress, sleep deprivation, overmedication with central nervous system depressants, or too much alcohol can diminish a person's ability to recall memories.

Agnosia

Agnosia describes a person's inability to recognize familiar memory patterns due to a disruption of the memory process, even though the person has fully functional sensory capabilities.

Damage to the cortical areas adjacent to the primary cortical centers for touch, vision, hearing, and smell will disrupt stored memories acquired through the sensory system. For example, lesions of the postcentral gyrus will interfere with the recognition of familiar objects identified through touch. Damage to the visual realm (an area neighboring the primary visual cortex) will impair the ability to recognize familiar objects, even though the patient's visual senses are intact.

Amnesia

Amnesia, simply defined as a loss of memory, can be psychogenic or organic in nature. People diagnosed with amnesia usually have impaired long-term memory. Specifically, patients with amnesia have severely impaired explicit memory performance, but show normal implicit memory performance on many tasks.

> Amnesia can be *anterograde,* in which there is an inability to form new memories, or *retrograde,* in which previous memories are not remembered.

Posttraumatic amnesia occurs following a severe head injury, and the duration of amnesia correlates with the severity of the injury. Retrograde amnesia is evident, usually affecting memories of events that occurred prior to the head injury.

Alzheimer Disease

Alzheimer disease is a well-known condition that is prevalent in the elderly.

> The initial symptoms may be manifest as minor forgetfulness, but progress to serious memory loss.

Although both explicit and implicit forms of memory are impaired in patients with Alzheimer disease, explicit memory is more seriously compromised. Patients are better at procedural memories, even though their declarative memories are diminished. In patients, memory loss may or may not be accompanied by various degrees of confusion, depression, restlessness, hallucinations, delusions, and disturbances in eating and sleeping behaviors.

β-Amyloid protein deposits (tangles and plaques) are characteristically found in the brains of deceased patients with Alzheimer disease. Associated with the β-amyloid deposits is atrophy of important brain regions, most notably the cerebral cortex, hippocampus, entorhinal cortex, and the basal forebrain—regions critical for memory formation and long-term storage. There is considerable controversy as to whether amyloid deposition is a cause of or an effect of the Alzheimer disease process.

Brain Trauma

Hippocampal Damage   The case of H.M. provides insight into the critical role of the hippocampus in forming new memories. People suffering from hippocampal damage (perhaps as a result of a cerebral infarct or trauma) will recall established memories but may not readily learn and retain new information. These patients retain the ability to form new procedural memories, even though the ability to form new long-term declarative memories is substantially diminished.

Frontal Cortical Lobe Damage   Patients with frontal lobe injury typically exhibit apathy, confusion, and memory impairment. Patients have great difficulty in recalling a temporal series of events, such as describing their life history starting from childhood to the present.

Genetic Influences on Learning and Memory

> Several genetic defects cause alterations in signal-transduction mechanisms, with serious consequences to the developing brain.

Severe mental retardation, among other physiological and anatomical abnormalities, is characteristic of Rubenstein–Taybi and Coffin–Lowry syndromes. Both syndromes directly or indirectly involve faulty CREB activity. CREB is involved in regulation of gene transcription. Cretinism is severe retardation caused by thyroid hormone (T_3) deficiency during a critical period of brain development. Under normal conditions, thyroid hormone binds to nuclear thyroid receptors, which contribute to transcriptional regulation.

Wernicke–Korsakoff Syndrome

Wernicke–Korsakoff syndrome commonly afflicts persons with a prolonged history of severe addiction to alcohol. Such individuals are nutritionally malnourished and develop thiamine (vitamin B_1) deficiency. Lack of vitamin B_1 results in impaired neuronal utilization of glucose. In Wernicke–Korsakoff syndrome a prolonged thiamine deficiency leads to a shrinkage or loss of neurons in various brain regions, particularly the hypothalamic mamillary bodies and the dorsomedial thalamus, which projects to the prefrontal cortex. Patients diagnosed with Wernicke–Korsakoff syndrome have neurological deficits similar to patients with frontal cortical lobe damage, and are likely to suffer from retrograde and anterograde amnesia.

OVERVIEW

At a cognitive level, memory can be classified into many different forms. Important, on-going research focuses on understanding the neurobiological processes that may underlie the many forms of memory. The primary competing hypotheses, synaptic versus neurochemical signal transduction, differ in terms of where the memories are stored—synaptic storage versus intracellular storage. However, both hypotheses share a common mechanism: increased intracellular calcium initiates events leading to augmented gene expression and de novo protein synthesis. The details of which genes are altered and which proteins are synthesized remain unknown. The burning question of the new millennium is whether LTP, neurochemical signal-transduction mechanisms, or some other hypothesis will be the "stuff that memories are made of."

Also unanswered is the intriguing question of how and why memories degrade. More than likely, continued research will reveal the cleverness and sophistication of Mother Nature: the cellular and molecular mechanisms underlying neuronal information storage will be shown to involve an integrated contribution of synaptic and neuronal signal-transduction responses. Moreover, understanding the mechanisms of memory will shed light on diseases and conditions that affect human memory. Elucidation of critical molecular targets that pathologically alter processes of memory will provide new insights for discovery of new drugs and therapeutic treatments. The future bodes an exciting, fascinating, and perhaps surprising destiny for neurobiological research on the processes of learning and memory.

· C H A P T E R · 1 3 ·

VIRAL EFFECTS ON NEURONS

·

Arlene R. Collins

Introduction

The Virus-Infected Cell

Host Responses to Virus Infection

Virus Entry into the CNS

Mechanisms of Neuropathogenesis

How Virus Infections Change Behavior and Learning

Viruses in Gene Therapy

Summary

· · · · · · · · · · · ·

INTRODUCTION

Viral infections that allow entry of the virus into the central nervous system (CNS) can cause damage to the brain, resulting in deterioration of cognitive and motor functioning.

How does a virus selectively damage the brain so as to alter only specific functions and not others? To answer this question it is necessary to consider the unique characteristics of CNS infections by viruses. How do viruses enter the brain? What immunological characteristics of the CNS protect the virus from elimination? What mechanisms do viruses use to alter the functioning of neurons in the CNS? Knowing how this works, what motivates scientists to continue to experiment with the use of viruses for gene therapy for disorders of the brain such as Parkinson and Alzheimer diseases?

Viruses as pathogens in the CNS are an attractive model for study. They have a limited number of genes that become amplified during virus replication. The products of viral gene expression can be readily detected by electron microscopy, immunofluorescence, and reverse transcription–polymerase chain reaction assay. An association between the presence of virus and the disease state can be made, and frequently the virus-induced disease can be adapted to an animal model.

The following definitions are useful in understanding viruses as pathogens in the CNS.

Neurotropism refers to the ability of the virus to infect CNS cells. *Neuroinvasion* is the ability of the virus to invade the CNS from the periphery. *Neurovirulence* is the ability of the virus to cause damage to the CNS.

THE VIRUS-INFECTED CELL

The viral life cycle takes place in a living cell and proceeds according to a one-step growth curve (Figure 13–1).

Infection is initiated by receptor-mediated adsorption of the virus to the cell surface followed by penetration through the plasma membrane by fusion or endocytosis and then uncoating to remove the protective protein coat and free the viral genome (genetic material).

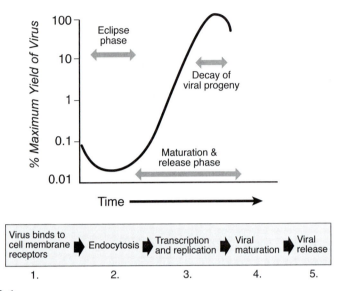

Figure 13–1
The one-step growth curve takes place in a living cell and has five separate events that generally occur. 1. The virus is adsorbed to cells via specific receptors. 2. The virus penetrates the cell by fusion or receptor-mediated endocytosis. 3. In the eclipse phase, transcription of viral messenger RNA and replication of the genome occur. 4 and 5. The maturation and release of progeny virus are the final intracellular events.

An eclipse phase then commences during which the viral genome directs synthesis of new viral DNA, RNA, and proteins. No infectious viral progeny can be detected until the maturation and release phase. During this phase the components that have accumulated in the eclipse phase are simultaneously assembled in large numbers and released from the cell in a single burst, often leading to lysis and death of the infected cell in a process called *lytic infection*. However, not all virus infections are lytic. Some viruses possess characteristics that favor a persistent replication strategy and cell sparing. These viruses have generated viral variants that are defective and cell sparing, or carry single or limited amino acid mutations that result in diminished expression of a viral gene product essential for viral replication. Persistent infection often occurs without disease.

HOST RESPONSES TO VIRUS INFECTION

Host responses are directed toward elimination of the virus.

The mononuclear phagocyte system responds by chemotaxis toward the site of infection and actively ingests and digests viruses and cell debris. Viral antigen stimulates B lymphocytes to produce antibodies that neutralize infectious virus and together with complement cause lysis of infected cells often before infectious viral progeny are made. Serum proteins that compose the complement system combine with antibody–viral complexes to enhance the elimination of virus and virus-infected cells. Effector T-lymphocyte responses are evoked by viral antigen and by cytokine stimulation. Viral antigen present on the infected cell in the context of major histocompatibility complex (MHC) class I and class II molecules is recognized by specific T cells that are capable of eliminating the infected cell. Finally, memory T and B cells are formed that act as sentinels to respond quickly to a repeat appearance of the virus.

Viruses that are successful pathogens have evolved mechanisms to evade host immune responses.

For example, human immunodeficiency virus (HIV) and influenza virus undergo mutations in the virus surface proteins so as to cause antigenic variation and escape from immune recognition. Viruses such as measles virus down-regulate expression of viral antigen on the infected cell surface. HIV infects cells of the immune system, for example, macrophages and T cells, leading to abrogation of immune functions. HIV and herpes virus sequester DNA copies of the viral genome inside the cell nucleus. In addition to evading host response, infected cells may become persistently infected if cell death is avoided. Such persistently infected cells may maintain normal metabolic function, but the virus may induce disorders in differentiated or so-called luxury functions such as synthesis of growth factors and endocrine secretion, which can lead to disturbances in brain homeostasis.

VIRUS ENTRY INTO THE CNS

The process of gaining access to the CNS, that is, *neuroinvasion,* is determined by the host's susceptibility to the virus and exists primarily at the level of the presence or absence of receptors for the virus.

Neurotropic viruses are viruses that have adapted to utilize neural cell surface molecules as receptors. The CNS is highly suited to virus adaptation and persistence. Restriction to entry of viruses is an innate property of the neuroectoderm. However, having once gained entry, a virus can rapidly disseminate through the

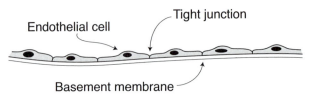

Figure 13–2
Many constituents of the plasma are unable to pass from the circulatory system into the CNS. The brain capillary endothelial cells, which are bound by tight junctions, and their supporting basement membrane form a blood–brain barrier. Perivascular astrocyte foot processes are in close contact with the basement membrane and play a less important role as a barrier.

complex network of neural interconnections. The brain capillary endothelial cells that are bound by tight junctions and their supporting basement membrane form a blood–brain barrier that restricts trafficking of antibodies, cytokines, monocyte/macrophages, and nonactivated lymphocytes into the brain (Figure 13–2). The CNS endothelial cell layer changes when activated by cytokines. A variety of selectins and adhesion molecules become expressed on the endothelial cell surface and provide the necessary receptors to attract immune cells. Tight junctions become leaky, allowing entry of antibodies, cytokines, immune cells, and even viruses into the CNS. CNS astrocytes and oligodendrocytes express low levels of MHC class I molecules, and neurons appear to express no MHC class I or class II at all. MHC class II expression can be induced in astrocytes by cytokine stimulation. Stimulated astrocytes, in the presence of virus, produce an antigen-activated cytotoxicity. As a consequence of low MHC class I expression, specific cytotoxic T-lymphocyte recognition of infected brain cells, particularly neurons, is absent. Additionally, many viruses have evolved strategies to abort the antigen-processing pathway involving MHC class I or class II complex formation with antigen.

Other factors of the host such as age, immune status, and genetic predisposition influence neuroinvasion and neurotropism. Also, pathogenic viruses will provoke injury to neural cells at a target site and evade immune responses of the host in order to persist and cause sustained injury. Neurons are essential for the host's survival and are irreplaceable once destroyed.

Sites of Neuroinvasion

Neural Route

The direct *neural route* of CNS entry is used by several viruses including herpes and rabies viruses (Figure 13–3).

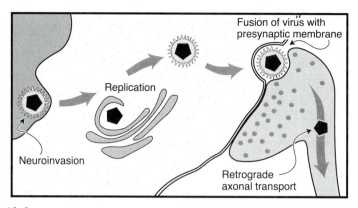

Figure 13–3

Direct neural entry and transneural passage of viruses. Viruses replicate in the cell nucleus and cytoplasm, traverse the endoplasmic reticulum, and acquire a membrane envelope as they bud through the Golgi apparatus into intracytoplasmic vesicles. Transneural passage occurs after fusion of the viral envelope with the postsynaptic membrane. The nucleocapsid undergoes retrograde axonal transport toward the cell body. [From K.L. Tyler and B.N. Fields, Pathogenesis of viral infections, in B.N. Fields, D.M. Knipe, and P.M. Howley (eds.): *Fields Virology*, 3d ed. New York: Lippincott-Raven, 1996; p. 173, with permission.]

These viruses enter peripheral neurons by fusion (herpes) or receptor-mediated endocytosis (rabies) and use fast intraaxonal retrograde transport, calculated to be 2–16 mm/day, to reach the temporal lobes (herpes) or limbic system (rabies). Neural transport of viruses can be prevented by nerve ablation or impeded by drugs that disrupt the microtubules, such as colchicine. The virus is released basolaterally at the postsynaptic terminals. The presynaptic terminals of nerve cells may contain increased numbers of virus receptors. Spread of viruses across synapses over linked interneural circuits between the peripheral and central nervous system transports the virus to the CNS, where further viral spread across linked interneural circuits occurs. Spread of viruses across synapses is not impeded by antibody responses in the host.

Hematogenous Route

To reach the CNS, blood-borne viruses must breach the blood–brain barrier.

Many viruses can either infect or be passively transported across capillary endothelial cells to invade the CNS. A particularly sparse basement membrane and fenestrated capillary endothelium occurs at the choroid plexus. Viruses that invade at this site enter the cerebrospinal fluid (CSF). Once in the CSF, viruses can infect ependymal cells lining the walls of the ventricles and then can invade the underlying brain tissue. A third mode of hematogenous entry is by trans-endothelial transport via diapedesis of infected monocytes, leukocytes, or lympho-cytes. This process, often referred to as the Trojan horse mechanism, may be modulated by viral activation of cell surface adhesion molecules. Vascular per-meability factors may facilitate viral neuroinvasion.

MECHANISMS OF NEUROPATHOGENESIS

When a virus causes neuropathology, the disease is associated with the presence of the virus at or near the target organ in the CNS.

Elicitation of the disease is associated with molecular and genetic determi-nants of neurovirulence. Viral structural and nonstructural proteins may be directly toxic to neurons. They also stimulate cytokine production. Cytokines released by local immune responses play an important role in neurotoxicity. They participate in the common pathway leading to neurotoxicity, that is, production of nitric oxide (NO) by astrocytes. NO facilitates excitatory injury to neurons through release of glutamate, often acting on N-methyl-D-aspartate (NMDA) receptors.

Glycoprotein G and Rabies Virus Neurovirulence

Glycoprotein G is an important determinant of rabies virulence (Figure 13–4).

Mutations in glycoprotein G cause the virus to spread more slowly and to lose the capacity to invade certain cells. Glycoprotein G binds to nicotinic acetylcholine (ACh) receptors. The synaptic terminals at the myoneural junction may contain increased numbers of receptors that facilitate transsynaptic spread of virus from

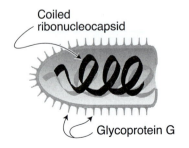

Figure 13–4
Schematic diagram of the bullet-shaped rabies virus showing the internal coiled ribonucleocapsid and the external surface of repeating units of the G envelope glycoprotein, which is responsible for attachment of the virus to receptors on susceptible cells.

infected myocytes to sensory neurons. Rabies virus also binds to cells that do not have ACh, using CD56, the neural cell adhesion molecule (NCAM), as receptor. Pathogenesis of rabies is dependent on major variations in glycoprotein G. The *street virus* strain of rabies is highly virulent, causing an encephalitic form of disease manifested as "furious" behavior in animals; *challenge virus* strain of rabies has low virulence, causing paralysis and manifested as "dumb" behavior in animals.

Human Immunodeficiency Virus (HIV) Glycoprotein 160: Neurotoxicity and Long-Term Potentiation

Glycoprotein 160 (gp160) is composed of two subunits: gp120 and gp41.

Gp120, the external domain responsible for recognition of the receptor, dissociates from the virus after attachment. Gp41 contains a fusion domain (F), a transmembrane domain, and a cytoplasmic tail (Figure 13–5). Gp120 binds to

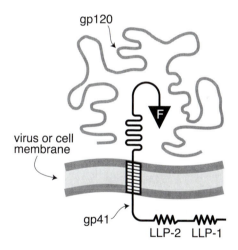

Figure 13–5
Human immunodeficiency virus (HIV) envelops glycoprotein, gp160, on the virus or cell surface. Viral gp160 is responsible for attachment of the virus to receptors on susceptible cells. Gp160 is produced as a precursor in infected cells and is cleaved intracellularly into gp120 and gp41 subunits. Gp120 is positioned on the external surface of the virus or cell membranes. Gp41 traverses the lipid bilayer and has an external fusion peptide (F) and intracytoplasmic LLP-2 and LLP-1 *Lentivirus* lytic peptides. [From P.A. Luciw, Human immunodeficiency viruses and their replication, in B.N. Fields, D.M. Knipe, and P.M. Howley (eds.): *Fields Virology,* 3d ed. New York: Lippincott-Raven, 1996; p. 1881, with permission.]

the CD4 receptor present on T lymphocytes and monocytes or to galacto-ceramide, which is present on oligodendrocytes and some neurons. Spread of infection from cell to cell also occurs by fusion of plasma membranes and mixing of the cytoplasmic contents. Gp120 requires a secondary receptor for entry, the CCRK5 chemokine receptor, which is involved in cell activation. The cytoplasmic tail of gp41 contains a linear region of 28 amino acids referred to as the genus *Lentivirus* lytic peptides, LLP-2 and LLP-1, which form a structure similar to certain cation channels when inserted into the plasma membrane.

> Long-term potentiation (LTP) is a target of HIV neurovirulence.

The mediator of disruption of LTP is gp160. The gp120 domain binds to the postsynaptic membrane, and the gp41 domain is inserted. The *Lentivirus* lytic peptides, LLP-2 and LLP-1, then form a cation channel that alters calcium flux, causing disruption of intracellular calcium homeostasis (Figure 13–6). As a result, postsynaptic calcium fails to rise, Ca^{2+}/calmodulin-dependent kinases are not activated, and the retrograde signals back to the presynaptic terminal are not generated. Therefore the persistent enhancement of transmitter release and LTP does not occur. LTP is a cellular mechanism associated with the formation of learning and memory that occurs in the cerebral cortex and hippocampus (see Chapter 12).

HOW VIRUS INFECTIONS CHANGE BEHAVIOR AND LEARNING

Infected neurons may respond to the presence of virus by altering their "luxury" functions, that is, those functions associated with terminally differentiated cells. As a consequence, higher mental functions are affected.

Rabies and the Hypothalamus

> In the early phase of rabies, there is selectivity of infection for neurons of the limbic system.

Characteristically, the hippocampus is a target organ. Infected neurons remain intact but are functionally disturbed. At this stage, rabid animals show behavioral disturbances characterized by severe agitation, disorientation, and hypersalivation. Such animals may initiate biting attacks on other wildlife or on humans. The stimuli for these oral tendencies arise abnormally in the amygdala and the medial region of the hypothalamus. James Papez, in 1937, proposed a

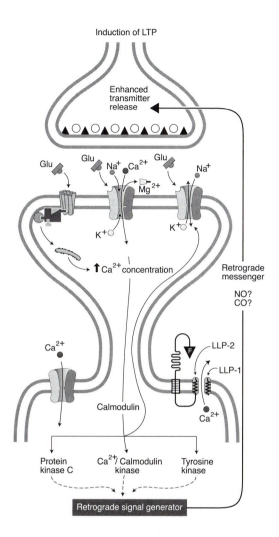

Figure 13–6

When the postsynaptic membrane is depolarized by the actions of non-NMDA receptor channels, as occurs during a high-frequency tetanus that induces long-term potentiation (LTP), the depolarization relieves the Mg^{2+} blockade of the NMDA channel. This allows Na^+, K^+, and Ca^{2+} to flow through the NMDA channel. The resulting rise in Ca^{2+} in the dendritic spine triggers calcium-dependent kinases (calcium/calmodulin kinase and kinase C), which induce LTP. Once LTP is induced, the postsynaptic cell releases a retrograde messenger that is thought to act on kinases in the presynaptic terminal to produce the sustained enhancement of neurotransmitter release that underlies the persistence of LTP. Insertion of gp41 into the postsynaptic membrane permits LLP-2 and LLP-1 domains to form a cation channel that alters Ca^{2+} flux. The disruption of intracellular calcium homeostasis will inhibit LTP. [From: Cellular mechanisms of learning and memory, in E.R. Kandel, J.H. Schwartz, and T.M. Jessell (eds.): *Essentials of Neural Science and Behavior.* Norwalk, CT: Appleton & Lange, 1995; p. 667, with permission.]

neural circuit for reciprocal communication between higher cortical centers and the hypothalamus. Papez' evidence was based on clinical observations that patients with rabies show profound changes in emotional state including bouts of terror and rage. The neural circuit he proposed is now called the *limbic system*. In this circuit, information from the associative cortex is processed through the cingulate gyrus to the hippocampus and the amygdala, which is then projected to the mamillary bodies of the hypothalamus. In turn, the hypothalamus provides information by a pathway from the mamillary bodies to the cingulate gyrus and the prefrontal cortex.

HIV and the Acquired Immunodeficiency Syndrome (AIDS) Dementia Complex

> AIDS dementia complex is commonly associated with HIV-infected patients not treated with antiviral agents and under conditions of profound immunosuppression.

The progressive loss of T lymphocytes and decreased immune activation of B lymphocytes and macrophages result in failure to control HIV replication and emergence of virus variants. Neurons and oligodendrocytes are a major target of the virus and undergo functional alteration in response to the persistent presence of the virus. Oligodendrocytes show myelin dysfunction that appears as white matter pallor on postmortem histopathological examination. Neurons survive but show progressive functional abnormalities.

> Clinical studies show that patients with AIDS dementia complex have progressive loss of cognitive abilities.

Specifically this includes attention, memory/learning, speech/language, abstraction/reasoning, and visuospatial skills. Patients have acquired abnormalities in motor function such as slowed movements, abnormal gait, limb incoordination, and poor manual dexterity. Concomitant with these symptoms, patients show a decline in motivation, emotional control, or change in social behavior such as apathy, inertia, irritability, and impaired judgment. Psychomotor speed tests such as Trail-Making, Grooved Pegboard, and Symbol Digit are most useful for screening for HIV dementia. A decline in CD4 T lymphocytes is related to a decline in performance on these tests. Other cognitive domains, such as language and attention, are often well preserved.

Pediatric HIV-associated CNS disease is most frequently manifest as developmental delays, cognitive impairment, and poor brain growth.

If in a progressive form, there is deterioration in social skills and loss of previously acquired language and adaptive skills. Most children show a more indolent form of deterioration. The rate of mental development declines as evidenced by a decline in IQ score. Motor ability is impaired, and there is poor brain growth. The clinical symptoms of HIV-associated CNS disease indicate that HIV compromises normal developmental processes. A better understanding of the underlying pathophysiological mechanisms is needed. Presynaptic facilitation or LTP is one target that HIV disrupts. Antiviral treatments that prevent HIV replication in the brain modulate and may even prevent this form of impairment.

VIRUSES IN GENE THERAPY

A goal of therapy for neurological disorders such as Parkinson disease and Alzheimer disease is restoration of normal function by replacement of lost or nonfunctional cells. Viruses may be used as vehicles for delivery of genes into the CNS to reintroduce a lost function to the surviving cells.

Nonreplicating virus vectors carry the gene of interest to the nucleus of the target neurons where it can be transcribed into the protein. A desirable goal is to provide long-term, regulated expression of the protein at therapeutic levels. A problem arises if an immune response to the vector is generated. This can lead to focal pathology and elimination of the vector-bearing cells.

Adenovirus as a Vector

The strategy for use of *adenovirus,* a DNA virus that is relatively non-cytopathic, is to substitute the foreign gene into the E1A region of the vector that is important for viral transcription.

Further deletions of genes from the vector are made in the E1B and E4 regions to relieve a block in host mRNA transport. However, use of this vector provided only transient expression of the transgene due to induction of a repressor that inactivated the promoter and due to loss of episomal vector DNA on cell division. Also, an inflammatory response due to virally induced cytokines was observed, but this response was not strong enough to eliminate transgene expression. Down-regulation of the immune response was aided by the adenovirus E3 gene, which disrupts MHC class I expression. Hence, although problems remain, these vectors show promise for gene therapy. Interaction of adenovirus vectors with receptors is subject to modification, and vectors that target cell populations more specifically can be expected. However, the Achilles heel of gene therapy is control of inflammation. One approach is to reduce antigenicity of the vector by further gene deletion. Another approach involves cytokine modulation. Vectors that are modified to carry additional genes for the synthesis of immunosuppressive cytokines are being investigated.

SUMMARY

Viruses infect and cause injury to the nervous system by specific mechanisms. Understanding these mechanisms is important for the development of methods to prevent and treat virus-induced neurological disorders.

Gene therapy using virus vectors may be an applicable mechanism to treat genetic diseases of the nervous system, to control malignant neoplasias, and to treat acquired degenerative encephalopathies (Alzheimer disease and Parkinson disease).

· I N D E X ·

NOTE: Page numbers in italics indicate figures; page numbers followed by *t* indicate tables.

NOTES

NOTES

NOTES

NOTES

NOTES

NOTES

NOTES

NOTES

NOTES

NOTES

NOTES

NOTES

NOTES

NOTES

NOTES

NOTES

NOTES

NOTES

NOTES